THE COUMADIN® COOKBOOK

A COMPLETE GUIDE *to* HEALTHY MEALS *when* TAKING COUMADIN®

RENE DESMARAIS, M.D.

GREGORY GOLDEN

GAIL BE

D1119747

THE COUMADIN® COOKBOOK

A COMPLETE GUIDE *to* HEALTHY MEALS *when* TAKING COUMADIN®

First Edition

RENE DESMARAIS, MD
GREGORY GOLDEN
GAIL BEYNON

Marsh Publishing Company
Salisbury, Maryland

COUMADIN® is a registered trademark of The Du Pont Merck Pharmaceutical Company

THE COUMADIN® COOKBOOK
A COMPLETE GUIDE *to* HEALTHY MEALS *when* TAKING COUMADIN®
By: RENE DESMARAIS, MD, GREGORY GOLDEN and GAIL BEYNON

Published by: MARSH PUBLISHING COMPANY
PO BOX 1597
SALISBURY, MD 21802-1597 USA

ISBN # 0-9664308-0-8

ATTENTION: SCHOOLS AND CORPORATIONS
MARSH books are available at quantity discounts with bulk purchase for educational, business, or sales promotional use. For information, please write to: Special Sales Department, Marsh Publishing Company, PO BOX 1597, Salisbury, MD 21802-1597

DISCLAIMERS

The use of COUMADIN® anticoagulants is always associated with some risk of morbidity and mortality. Although it is hoped that the use of this book will help some patients to regulate, more easily, their dose of COUMADIN® and their prothrombin time/INR, the authors can not and do not make any guarantee regarding these potential benefits. Also, the authors can not and do not guarantee any reduction in the risk associated with the use of COUMADIN® anticoagulants. The risks of COUMADIN® anticoagulants will not be eliminated by the use of this book and therefore the authors are not responsible for any complications, including death, that may result from COUMADIN® use. Consultation with the health professional or professionals responsible for prescribing the patient's COUMADIN® dose and monitoring the patient's prothrombin time/INR is necessary and strongly recommended before a change in the patient's diet. The responsibility for the risks associated with COUMADIN® use remain with the patient and the health professional or professionals described above. If the purchaser of this book does not wish to be bound by the above, the book may be returned to the publisher for a full refund.

The COUMADIN® Cook Book has not been endorsed by the DuPont Merck Pharmaceutical Company ("DuPont Merck"), nor has the information set forth in the COUMADIN® Cook Book been authorized or approved by DuPont Merck. DuPont Merck is not responsible for the accuracy of such information and expressly disclaims any responsibility to correct such information. In no event will DuPont Merck be liable for damages, including special, incidental, consequential, or indirect damages arising from the use of the COUMADIN® Cook Book, however caused and/or under any theory of liability. This limitation will apply even if DuPont Merck has been advised of the possibility of any such damage.

The Authors

RENÉ DESMARAIS MD currently practices Cardiology with Peninsula Cardiology Associates on the Eastern Shore of Maryland and in Delaware. His practice includes the largest COUMADIN® Clinic on the Delmarva Peninsula. He received his BA from The Johns Hopkins University in 1983. He graduated from The University of Connecticut Medical School, where he was a Scholar in Medicine, in 1987. From 1987 to 1990, he trained in internal medicine at Francis Scott Key Medical Center, now know as Bayview Medical Center, a hospital affiliated with The Johns Hopkins Hospital, in Baltimore. MD. Subsequently, he completed a Fellowship in Cardiovascular Diseases at The University of Virginia Medical Center in 1993. After this training he began practicing on the Eastern Shore where he lives with his wife, Cairy Packard, MD, and their three daughters. Dr. Desmarais' research has been published in *Circulation* and in the *Journal of The American College of Cardiology.*

GREGORY GOLDEN is a Cardiovascular Technologist with Peninsula Cardiology Associates on the Eastern Shore of Maryland. Greg spent seven years in the U.S. Navy. His spare time is taken by kayaking, cycling and Martial Arts.

GAIL BEYNON is an enthusiastic gardener and cook who began cooking at the age of five. Gail continues to experiment with new recipes and ingredients growing the produce in her garden when she can't find it locally. Despite 32 years as a full time computer specialist, Gail has developed a cooking data base with thousands of recipes. When she travels, Gail visits local grocery stores looking for unusual ingredients and new methods of preparation. While other folks may bring back artwork or jewelry, Gail brings home local foods and new recipe ideas to the enthusiastic reception of her family and friends.

Special thanks go to **Cairy Packard, MD**, **Jeffrey Beynon** and **Rita Murdock** for their meticulous editing of the final cookbook and Rita (Gail's mom) for letting her play in the kitchen at the age of five.

TABLE OF CONTENTS

DISCLAIMERS *3*

INTRODUCTION 21

USEFUL DIETARY TIPS FOR THE PATIENT ON COUMADIN® *27*

LIST OF FOODS WITH VERY LOW VITAMIN K CONTENT *31*

USEFUL INFORMATION FOR THE COOK 35

ODDS AND ENDS *36*

SUBSTITUTIONS *39*

ONE OUNCE (30 GRAMS) FOOD MEASURES *42*

MEASUREMENT CHART *43*

ONE POUND (450 GRAMS) FOOD MEASURES *44*

APPETIZERS 45

SHRIMP SPREAD 46

CHEDDAR-ALE CHEESE LOGS 46

AMARETTO CHEESE SPREAD 47

DRIED TOMATO SMOKY SPREAD 48

STUFFED MUSHROOMS 48

VERMONT CHEDDAR AND MAPLE CRACKERS 49

MIXED ANTIPASTO PLATTER 49

CRACKERS DEL PASEO 50

GARLICKY CLAM DIP 50

CRAB DIP 51

TANGY BLUE CHEESE DIP 51

ARTICHOKE DIP 52

GOLDEN CITRUS-RAISIN DIP 52

CAESAR MAYO DIP 53

TIPSY TUNA DIP 53

CAPONATA (EGGPLANT APPETIZER) 54

CRAB-MELT CANAPÉS 55

SALMON AND GOUDA PATE 56

DEVILED EGGS 57

CANTALOUPE FRUIT SALAD 57

SALMON MOUSSE 58

CARAMELIZED CARNITAS 59

GRILLED BRUSCHETTA WITH FRESH MOZZARELLA AND TOMATOES 60

BLACK CHERRY YOGURT CREAM DIP 60

EGGPLANT CAVIAR 61

CROSTINI A LA PORCINI 62

BREADS, SANDWICHES & SPREADS 63

CHEDDAR BISCUITS 64

GARDEN PIZZA 65

PIZZA DOUGH: 66

CHEDDAR FANS 67

MUFFINS: BASIC AND VARIATIONS 68

GINGER MUFFINS: 68

BANANA PECAN MUFFINS: 68

BLUEBERRY MUFFINS: 68

ORANGE MUFFINS: 69

CHEESE MUFFINS: 69

SURPRISE MUFFINS: 69

BUTTERMILK BISCUITS 69

QUICK AND EASY ROLLS 70

EGG PANCAKES 70

DATE OR RAISIN BRAN MUFFINS 71

CORN MEAL MUFFINS 72

RICE PANCAKES 72

BACON AND ONION MUFFINS 73

SAUSAGE, EGGPLANT, BASIL AND TOMATO PIZZA 74

JUMBO POPOVERS 75

SMOKED SALMON-AND-CHIVE SANDWICHES 75

ORANGE SPREAD 76

TUNA BUNS 76

EARLY BIRD BUTTERMILK PANCAKES 77

BLUEBERRY BUTTERMILK PANCAKES 78

APPLE PANCAKE PUFF 79

GARLIC BREAD 80

POTATO CRACKERS 80

BASIC PANCAKES 81

SCOTTISH SCONES 82

IRISH SODA BREAD 83

APPLESAUCE BANANA BREAD 84

BEEF 85

BEEF STIR FRY 86

BEEF STROGANOFF 87

MEATLOAF 88

BREADED VEAL CUTLET (WEINERSCHNITZEL) 88

BEEF TACOS 89

CROCK POT CHILI CON CARNE 90

HAMBURG CASSEROLE 90

TEXAS CHILI 91

ENCHILADA PIE 92

VEAL PARMIGIANA 93

VEAL MARSALA 94

VEAL NORMANDE 94

SAUCY MEATLOAF 95

VEAL OSCAR WITH SHRIMP 96

VEAL CHILI 97

VEAL PICCATA 98

VEAL SCALOPPINI 99

OVEN-BAKED BOURGUIGNONNE 100

STEAK PARMIGIANA 101

VEAL SALTIMBOCCA A LA ROMANA 102

ITALIAN MEAT LOAF 103

UPSIDE DOWN PIZZA 104

GARLIC MEATBALLS 106

POULTRY 107

CHICKEN RAGOUT 108

CHICKEN-FILLED TORTILLAS 109

CROCKPOT BAKED CHICKEN BREASTS 109

JAMAICAN JERK CHICKEN 110

QUICK CHICKEN CREOLE 110

CHICKEN GUMBO 111

SAUCY HAM AND CHICKEN 112

RASPBERRY CHICKEN BREASTS 113

LEMON ONION CHICKEN 113

CHICKEN BREASTS DIANE 114

CHICKEN PICCATA 115

TURKEY SPAGHETTI SAUCE 115

CHICKEN BREASTS WITH DRIED BEEF 116

MARSALA CHICKEN BREASTS 117

SAUTÉ CHICKEN BREAST WITH MUSHROOMS 118

CHICKEN SAUTÉ BOURGUIGNONNE 119

ROAST TURKEY 120

LAMB 121

OVEN-COOKED LAMB STEW 122

GREEK-ROAST LEG OF LAMB 123

LEG OF LAMB 124

CROWN ROAST OF LAMB 124

MUSTARD & WINE MARINATED LAMB CHOPS 126

ARTILLERY RACK OF LAMB 126

ATHENIAN LAMB STEW 127

GRILLED LAMB AND SAUSAGE KEBABS 128

PORK 129

PEACHY PORK CHOPS 130

PORK CHOPS BRAISED WITH CIDER AND APPLES 130

NEAPOLITAN PORK CHOPS 131

BAKED PORK CHOPS 132

GLAZED PORK LOIN ROAST 132

LEMON PECAN PORK CHOPS 133

PORK PINWHEELS WITH APRICOT STUFFING 134

BAKED HAM WITH PINEAPPLE 135

GRILLED BRATWURST 136

PEANUT PORK CHOPS 136

PORK CHOPS WITH ONIONS 137

GRILLED PORK TENDERLOIN WITH MUSTARD CREAM 138

MUSHROOM SAUSAGE PIE 139

HAM IN ZIPPY CREAM SAUCE 140

HAM AND CHEESE PIE 140

PORK LOIN WITH MUSTARD CRUST 141

PORK MARENGO 143

PORK CHOPS IN TOMATO SAUCE WITH OREGANO 144

SEAFOOD 145

SAUTÉED GARLIC SHRIMP 146

PAN FRIED TUNA 146

PEPPER GRILLED SALMON 147

BAKED FISH 148

MEDITERRANEAN BAKED FISH 149

ARTICHOKE BOTTOMS WITH SHRIMP SAUTÉ 150

SALMON GRILL DIABLE 151

SHRIMP WITH TOMATO SAUCE 152

SEAFOOD STROGANOFF 153

BALSAMIC-GLAZED SALMON FILLETS 154

SCALLOPED OYSTERS 155

SALMON WITH PISTACHIO-BASIL BUTTER 156

BAKED SALMON WITH FETA VINAIGRETTE 157

GRILLED FISH IN FOIL 158

EGGS & CHEESE 159

SAUSAGE & EGG CASSEROLE 160

SCOTCH EGGS 161

BRUNCH ENCHILADAS 162

ITALIAN EGGS 163

SPICY BREAKFAST SAUSAGE CASSEROLE 164

SOUPS 165

GAZPACHO 166

GOULASH SOUP 166

SHERRIED CHICKEN SOUP 167

OLD-FASHIONED CHICKEN SOUP 168

CHICKEN AND RICE SOUP 168

CHICKEN SOUP 169

BAKED POTATO CHICKEN SOUP- 170

ITALIAN VEGETABLE SOUP WITH PROSCIUTTO 171

TOMATO-BEEF SOUP 172

TEX-MEX BEEF SOUP 173

VEGETABLE-BEEF SOUP 174

CREAMY BEEF-NOODLE COMBO 174

RED FISH CHOWDER 175

SOPA DE PESCADO (FISH) 176

GREEN CHILE SAUCE 176

QUICK FISH CHOWDER 177

TOMATO BISQUE 178

CARROT VICHYSSOISE 178

VEGETABLE SOUP 179

BEEF AND LENTIL STEW 180

PUREE OF CARROT SOUP 180

CARROT HORSERADISH SOUP 181

CARROT POTATO CHOWDER 182

SAUSAGE CHOWDER 182

CORN CHOWDER 183

MUSHROOM SOUP 184

BEAN SOUP 185

WHITE GAZPACHO 186

STRAW MUSHROOM SOUP 186

POTATO SOUP 187

SWEET SQUASH BISQUE 188

FRUIT SOUP 188

TOMATO SOUP 189

FRENCH ONION SOUP 190

HUNGARIAN STYLE SOUP 191

HEARTY CHICKEN AND RICE SOUP 192

MINESTRONE SOUP 192

WINTER SQUASH, APPLE AND WALNUT SOUP 193

GOLDEN MUSTARD SQUASH SOUP 194

RICE PASTA & POTATOES 195

TASTY WHITE RICE WITH CORN 196

BAKED POTATOES STUFFED WITH COTTAGE CHEESE 196

RAW POTATO LOAF 197

MACARONI AND CHEESE 197

PASTA AND TURKEY MEAT RED SAUCE 198

MEAT PASTA SAUCE 199

MY RICE-A-RONI 200

QUICK TOMATO SAUCE FOR PASTA 200

POLENTA 201

SHRIMP AND WINE-SAUCED SPAGHETTI 202

PASTA JAMBALAYA 203

POLISH NOODLES AND CABBAGE 204

HERBED RICE TOSS 205

CHEESY RICE AND HAM 206

CANDIED SWEET POTATOES 206

LEMON HERB ROASTED POTATOES 207

POTATO CASSEROLE 208

VEGETABLES 209

SMOTHERED GREENS 210

LIMA BEANS AND SPINACH 210

VEGETABLE STEW 211

SUCCOTASH 211

MAPLE WHIPPED BUTTERNUT SQUASH 212

STUFFED ARTICHOKES 212

BALSAMIC SQUASH PUREE 213

SUMMER SQUASH STIR-FRY 214

STRING BEANS, SOUTHERN STYLE 214

FRIED GARLIC GREEN BEANS 215

BABY CARROTS GLAZED WITH BUTTER 216

CAULIFLOWER PANCAKES 216

ZUCCHINI AND CHEDDAR BAKE 217

CAULIFLOWER WITH TOMATOES 217

STUFFED PEPPERS 218

ZUCCHINI CASSEROLE 218

ZUCCHINI-TOMATO PIE 219

BASQUE PEPPER STEW 220

BEST EVER BAKED BEANS 220

ONION PANCAKES 221

LEMON VEGGIES 222

PINEAPPLE YAM BAKE 222

COOKIES 223

RUGALA 224

PUMPKIN BARS WITH CREAM CHEESE FROSTING 225

CREAM CHEESE FROSTING 226

MEXICAN WEDDING COOKIES 226

CHOCOLATE WALNUT SQUARES 227

BROWN BUTTER ICING 228

PEANUT BUTTER COOKIES 228

FUDGE BROWNIES 229

CHOCOLATE FROSTING: 230

RAISIN-FILLED BARS 231

ALMOND BUTTER COOKIES 232

SOUR CREAM COOKIES 232

CAKES 233

MARBLE CHEESECAKE 234

FRUIT COCKTAIL CAKE 235

CHEESECAKE 236

PUMPKIN-RAISIN CAKE 237

GOLDEN FRUITCAKE 238

TANGERINE POUND CAKE 239

APPLE CAKE 240

RASPBERRY WALNUT CAKE 241

ANGEL FOOD CAKE 242

CHOCOLATE PUDDING CAKE 243

APPLE COFFEE CAKE 244

RAINBOW CAKES 245

FUZZY NAVEL CHEESECAKE 246

ORANGE MARMALADE GLAZE 246

CARROT/ZUCCHINI/APRICOT/PINEAPPLE CAKE 248

CRANBERRY SWIRL CHEESECAKE 250

HUNGARIAN COFFEE CAKE 251

GLAZED BLUEBERRY SHORTCAKE 252

CHOCOLATE HAZELNUT TORTE 253

DARK RUM GLAZE 254

SEVEN MINUTE COFFEE FROSTING 254

BISCUIT SHORTCAKE 255

SEVEN MINUTE FROSTING 256

DESSERTS 257

BAKED PEARS IN WINE 258

KIWI FRUIT ICE 258

FRUITY BREAD PUDDING 259

FRUIT COCKTAIL TORTE 260

STRAWBERRIES NAPOLEAN 260

CREME TOPPING 262

FUDGE SAUCE 262

WHIPPED CREAM 263

VANILLA SAUCE 264

TART APRICOT SAUCE 265

PEACH MELBA TRIFLE 266

CHOCOLATE BREAD PUDDING 267

PEPPERED STRAWBERRIES 268

PIES 269

PIE CRUST 270

SWEET POTATO PIE 270

PUMPKIN PIE 271

FUDGE PECAN PIE 272

CREAM RAISIN PIE 273

BANANA CREAM PIE 273

QUICK & EASY APPLE PIE 274

SALADS, DRESSINGS & SAUCES 275

LETTUCE SALAD 276

ELBOW MACARONI WITH GRAPES 276

TOMATO AND CABBAGE SALAD 276

PIZZA STYLE TOMATO SALAD 277

CUMIN FLAVORED CARROT SALAD 278

ITALIAN MARINATED TOMATOES 278

PINEAPPLE COLESLAW 279

GREEN BEANS CAESAR 280

CUCUMBER "NOODLES" WITH TOMATO SALSA 281

TOMATO AND CUCUMBER SALAD 282

HOLLANDAISE SAUCE 282

EASY BEARNAISE SAUCE 283

BERNAISE SAUCE 283

HAND-MADE MAYONNAISE 284

BASIC BLENDER MAYONNAISE 285

ANOTHER BLENDER MAYONNAISE 285

TOFU MAYONNAISE 286

VINEGAR & ONION SALAD DRESSING 286

CAJUN MAYONNAISE 287

SALSA 287

BASIC VINAIGRETTE 288

BALSAMIC VINAIGRETTE DRESSING 288

WHITE SAUCE 289

CHEDDAR CHEESE SAUCE 289

MUSHROOM CREAM SAUCE 289

SAVORY WHITE SAUCE 290

ITALIAN HERB DRESSING 290

GREEK SALAD DRESSING 291

HONEY MUSTARD SALAD DRESSING 291

CURTIDO SALVADORENO 292

BEVERAGES 293

SUMMER FRUIT BLEND 294

ORANGE JULIUS TYPE DRINK 294

FRUIT SMOOTHIE 295

CIDER SNAP 295

HOT BUTTERED RUM 296

MULLED CIDER 296

BLONDE SANGRIA 297

STRAWBERRY SHAKE 297

PUNCH 298

RED SANGRIA 298

INDEX 299

TEAR OUT - LIST OF FOODS WITH VERY LOW VITAMIN K CONTENT 315

TEAR OUT - LIST OF FOODS WITH VERY LOW VITAMIN K CONTENT 317

INTRODUCTION

by René Desmarais, MD

Welcome to the COUMADIN® Cookbook!

The goal of this cookbook is to allow the person on COUMADIN® to EASILY consume approximately the same amount of vitamin K each day in a heart-healthy way. This is essential for maintaining a PT/INR (prothrombin time/International Normalized Ratio) within the desired therapeutic range on a given COUMADIN® dose. The cookbook provides practical dietary guidelines for patients who take the anticoagulant COUMADIN®. Patients who take the generic form of COUMADIN®, warfarin sodium, can also use this cookbook. We intend to provide these guidelines in an enjoyable manner, primarily by furnishing the reader with recipes that are tasty, heart healthy, contain all food groups (including plenty of vegetables) and contain an accurate estimate of vitamin K content.

We want these guidelines to be easy to use and to understand. There are four major parts to this cookbook. The first part is this part, the introduction. The second part gives several useful tips on how to consume a more steady or consistent daily amount of vitamin K. The third part is a list of foods that contain very small amounts of vitamin K. The fourth part is the recipes themselves. Every food, drink and recipe included in this cookbook has a known amount of vitamin K per serving. So, by using all four parts of the cookbook, the patient on COUMADIN® can eat approximately the same amount of vitamin K every day AND have an enjoyable, healthy diet.

The amount of vitamin K that the patient on COUMADIN® consumes each day is crucial to keep the effect of COUMADIN® steady. COUMADIN® works to increase the time it takes for a patient's blood to clot by going against the action of vitamin K. By doing this, COUMADIN® PREVENTS harmful blood clots from forming. Likewise, vitamin K goes against the action of COUMADIN®. Vitamin K HELPS blood clot. Therefore, if patients do not consume a steady amount of vitamin K each day, while they are taking COUMADIN®, they are in danger of their blood forming unwanted clots too quickly or of prolonged bleeding from too much drug effect. By using this cookbook, the person on COUMADIN® may have a more stable effect from his or her COUMADIN® dose. Also, a more stable COUMADIN® dose may lead to fewer prothrombin time/INR tests (the prothrombin time test is the blood test that your health care professional uses to monitor the effects of COUMADIN®).

Before we proceed, it is necessary to make certain that all of our readers understand some basics about the use of the anticoagulant COUMADIN®. An anticoagulant is simply any drug that prevents blood from clotting as well as it should. Not all anticoagulants are COUMADIN®. The generic name for COUMADIN® is warfarin sodium. COUMADIN®, a trademark name belonging to The DuPont Merck Pharmaceutical Company, is the most commonly used warfarin sodium product in the U.S. today. Aspirin and heparin are drugs that also affect the blood's ability to form clots, but these products are not affected by vitamin K. COUMADIN® opposes the action of vitamin K in the body. One of the most important actions of vitamin K is to help the liver make proteins that circulate in our blood and cause blood to clot. These proteins are not the only things in our blood that make blood clot in the appropriate circumstances. Aspirin, for example, makes blood less likely to clot because it opposes blood cells called platelets. Platelets also help make blood clot, but platelets are not affected by COUMADIN®.

The typical patient on COUMADIN® receives contradictory advice regarding their diet. Often they are told to avoid foods with high vitamin K content so that vitamin K will not antagonize the effect of COUMADIN®. They are told this so their dose of COUMADIN® can be more easily managed. Further, they are told to "eat the same amount" of a given food each day, for example "You can eat spinach, but you have to have EXACTLY the same amount each day." This is very difficult to do in real life. Finally, the major food group they are told to avoid is vegetables. However, most, if not all, heart healthy dietary guidelines strongly emphasize the need to have a large amount of vegetables in the diet. So then, how does the average patient on COUMADIN® reconcile all of these inconsistent recommendations? The answer is simply that they often cannot. Thus, we hope to provide more practical guidelines to these patients, their loved ones, and their caregivers, if applicable.

If you have read this far, then you may be interested in this cookbook because you or a loved one has had a conversation like this with a physician or other health care professional:

DR: Hello Mr. or Ms. COUMADIN® Patient. Are you enjoying your supper? We have determined that you have blankety-blank (fill-in your particular diagnosis). This disorder requires that you begin COUMADIN® therapy.

Patient: Oh, can you tell me what that means?

DR: Yes, of course. First of all, you will take COUMADIN® so that your blood will not clot too much. It means you will have to have a lab test called a prothrombin time/INR on a regular basis. The prothrombin time/INR tells us how COUMADIN® is working and allows your health care professional to keep you within a desired therapeutic range. You may not be able to eat some of your favorite foods. In addition, you need to do this while staying on a heart healthy diet.

Patient: So, what exactly can I eat, since I am trying to stick to a heart healthy diet?

DR: Well, there are lots of things you can eat. However, there are also quite a few foods you really should try to stay away from.

Patient: Such as?

DR: Green leafy vegetables, such as spinach, lettuce and so forth. Also, you should avoid other green vegetables, like asparagus, peas, brussel sprouts, broccoli, seaweed, and so forth. There are other guidelines, outlined in that small pamphlet we gave you.

Patient: But aren't those foods good for me?

DR: Yes, of course they are!

Patient: I'm sorry doctor, but I'm a little confused about what I should eat. Can you help me with the foods I can and should eat?

Unfortunately, the answer to the patient's last question is not simple. However, one point is simple: If you are a patient on COUMADIN®, with or without atherosclerosis, (atherosclerosis = cholesterol plaques in arteries of the body), you may think your dietary choices are limited. You can try to eat the same, small amount of foods high in vitamin K each day, but this is extremely difficult. Or, you can try to eat foods that contain only a little vitamin K, but this is difficult, also. Thus, to help the patient on COUMADIN® consume a steady (or consistent) amount of vitamin K on a daily basis, every recipe and individual food item in this cookbook will have an accurate estimate of its vitamin K content. Because of small differences in the amount of vitamin K that are present even in the same quantity of any given food item, the best we can attain at this point is an accurate estimate of the amount of vitamin K in any recipe or food item. Nonetheless, we believe such an estimate is far superior to no estimate at all and, therefore, can only help in keeping the COUMADIN® effect steady.

Another important bit of knowledge the reader should have is the actual amount of vitamin K in a typical diet. The average amount of vitamin K a person in the U.S. consumes per day is approximately 60 to 80 micrograms (mcgs). One microgram (mcg) is one- thousandth of a gram. Remember that twenty-nine (29) grams equal an ounce. Thus, you can see, we are talking about a tiny amount of vitamin K when we talk about the typical diet. Nonetheless, variations in small amounts of vitamin K can have a large effect on prothrombin time/INR in some patients.

As stated above, the patient on COUMADIN® is often instructed to limit the amount of vitamin K in his or her diet so as not to counteract the effect of the COUMADIN®. This advice has a few problems as regards the overall health of the patient. First, this leads to a decrease or entire lack in the consumption of many vegetables which provide many other essential nutrients and which are strongly recommended by most, if not all, heart healthy diets, including, for example, the DASH diet of the National Heart, Lung, and Blood Institute. Second, the importance and mechanism of action of vitamin K in tissues such as bone is not well known. The lack of vitamin K in these tissues could have unknown side effects for the individual on a low vitamin K diet. Third, the concept of a low vitamin K diet may not necessarily be the safest in terms of a

relatively consistent "desired" or therapeutic effect of the COUMADIN®
dose on a daily basis. More on this in the next paragraph.

    We are ready to make firm recommendations regarding the daily
intake of vitamin K in the diet of patients on COUMADIN®. As we have
said, the patient on COUMADIN® is told to either take in a small amount
of vitamin K daily, or to at least take in the same amount daily. But, if the
patient tries to take in a small amount of vitamin K each day, then the
patient can easily take in too much vitamin K by mistake. This would
make the patient's blood more likely to develop unwanted clots, which
could be dangerous. On the other hand, if the patient tries to take in the
same amount of vitamin K each day, this is very difficult without accurate
guidelines. This difficulty can cause the patient's blood to form unwanted
clots or cause prolonged bleeding. It is important to understand that the
typical patient on COUMADIN® does NOT need to STRICTLY limit his
or her vitamin K intake, but rather to take in an amount consistent with the
recommended daily allowance (RDA) in an ACCURATELY
ESTIMATED manner. Therefore, we recommend that the patient on
COUMADIN® uses the guidelines in this cookbook to try to take in
approximately 100 micrograms of vitamin K each day. This may not be
possible for every patient on COUMADIN®. Also, the intake of this
amount of vitamin K daily may not be beneficial for every patient taking
COUMADIN®. Each patient should, working with his or her doctor or
other health care provider, find their own best daily vitamin K intake and
use the guidelines in this book to keep their intake as steady as possible.
Finally, since this approach must always be undertaken only with thorough
understanding of the individual patient, we strongly recommend that the
patient always consult his or her doctor prior to ANY change in his or her
diet that may alter the COUMADIN® effect and laboratory test results.

    By using the vitamin K content of the recipes and individual food
items provided in this book, we hope that each reader can devise a diet on
a daily basis that will provide a steady and consistent amount of vitamin
K. This may be difficult, even if the vitamin K content of each individual
recipe or food is known. Thus, we strongly encourage every reader to
keep a diary. The diary should list the amount of vitamin K they have
consumed that day. The diary must be carefully kept. For example, with
each meal, the amount of vitamin K should be recorded in the diary, so

that the patient on COUMADIN® can aim for a constant amount of vitamin K each day. Finally, the reader can continue to use some of his or her own heart healthy recipes, if all the ingredients contain very small amounts of vitamin K. We have provided a list of foods with very low vitamin K content that the patient can use in his or her own recipes. It should be noted, however, that not ALL foods have well-established levels of vitamin K.

USEFUL DIETARY TIPS FOR THE PATIENT ON COUMADIN®

In addition to the recipes provided in this cookbook, there are several important facts regarding the vitamin K content of foods that should be mentioned. By following the tips outlined in this section, the patient on COUMADIN® can improve the stability of the amount of vitamin K in their diet and, hopefully, the stability of the effect of COUMADIN®.

1. The vitamin K content of vegetables varies depending on the location where they are grown. Thus, the patient on COUMADIN® has to be careful when traveling since the vitamin K content of vegetables in one part of the country may be different from vegetables in another part of the country. Unfortunately, at this time, there is no easy solution to this problem. Currently, we recommend that the patients use the estimates provided in this cookbook.

2. The vitamin K content of recipes that contain fresh vegetables only apply when fresh vegetables are used. The effect of canning or drying on the vitamin K content of vegetables is unknown at this time. Thus, when using this cookbook, the patient must only use fresh veggies, unless stated otherwise.

3. Some multivitamins contain vitamin K. This does not mean you cannot take these vitamins, it just means that you have to take into account their vitamin K content in your daily diary when you take them.

4. Dried basil, thyme, and oregano contain a high amount of vitamin K. However, a teaspoon of fresh basil, thyme, or oregano would be expected to contain very small amounts of vitamin K. Notice that recipes in this book only use fresh basil, thyme and oregano and they are used only in small quantities.

5. Store-bought mayonnaise, and margarine are VERY BAD. The reason? They contain unknown quantities of various vegetable oils and therefore the amount of vitamin K in these foods is unpredictable. They should be avoided altogether. Butter should be used instead of margarine. We have

provided recipes for homemade mayonnaise that contain a known quantity of vitamin K. Only homemade mayonnaise should be used.

6. Store-bought salad dressings may contain unknown quantities of various vegetable oils. They may also contain unknown quantities of herbs that are high in vitamin K. Some store-bought salad dressings have a low amount of vitamin K and are safe to use. However, identifying the store-bought salad dressings that are low in vitamin K can be very difficult for the patient on COUMADIN®, Therefore we have provided several recipes for homemade salad dressings that contain a known quantity of vitamin K.

7. Watch out for foods that should be low in vitamin K, but are packed in vegetable oils. Certain types of vegetable oils can contain high amounts of vitamin K and when the quantity of oil and/or type of oil is unknown, this can lead to large variations in vitamin K in the diet. The best example of this is tuna fish. This is an excellent food choice for the patient on COUMADIN®, since it is both heart healthy and very low in vitamin K WHEN IT IS EATEN FRESH OR WHEN IT IS PACKED IN WATER. However, tuna is often packed in oil, and then the vitamin K content is much higher and UNKNOWN! Therefore, only consume tuna (and other canned items) that are packed in water, NOT OIL.

8. Factors other than vitamin K intake can affect COUMADIN®. Illness can affect your prothrombin time/INR. Also, MANY medications, both prescription and over-the-counter, can affect your prothrombin time/INR. Remember that the prothrombin time/INR is a laboratory test used to monitor the effects of COUMADIN®. Therefore, you should always tell your doctor when you are sick or when you are starting or stopping a new medicine or when the dose of one of your medicines is changed.

9. Vitamin K content of food is not altered by cooking or gamma irradiation.

10. Exposure of oils to sunlight or fluorescent light destroys approximately 85% of the vitamin K. Several recipes included in this cookbook use Canola oil or olive oil (we chose these oils because they are heart healthy). The vitamin K content of these oils can be quite high. Therefore, before using these oils, you must first expose them to sunlight or fluorescent light for at least 48 hours. This will destroy the majority of vitamin K in the oils and decrease the variability of vitamin K in the diet. Interestingly, and distressingly, while researching this cookbook, we found wide variations in the amount of vitamin K levels reported to be present in various oils.

11. Beware of any food that contains vegetable oils in unknown quantities.

12. Fat in the diet is required for adequate vitamin K absorption. In fact, fat in the diet is required for the absorption of vitamins A, E and D as well. Thus, the use of VERY low fat diets is discouraged. Diets should contain approximately 25% fat.

13. The intake of large doses of vitamin E can affect the response of the body to vitamin K. Specifically, when taken in large doses, this vitamin may counteract the effect of vitamin K. Thus, intake of megadoses of vitamin E could further increase the patient's prothrombin time/INR and increase the effect of COUMADIN®. How vitamin E counteracts the effect of vitamin K is unknown. Thus, at this time, we can only recommend that a constant amount of this vitamin should be consumed on a daily basis. It would seem wise simply to take the RDA of this vitamin each day. However, the patient with coronary artery disease should consume 400 IU (international units) of vitamin E per day since this dose of vitamin E has been shown to have benefit in patients with coronary artery disease. There is no evidence that a constant intake of this amount of vitamin E per day would dangerously affect the prothrombin time/INR. However, we must again emphasize the importance of a constant amount of vitamin E.

14. NO GRAPEFRUIT or GRAPEFRUIT JUICE should be consumed by the patient on COUMADIN®!

15. BEWARE THE AVOCADO!! There are two reasons for this. First, the amount of vitamin K in avocado and avocado products such as guacamole can vary by as much as 40 times! Thus, the avocado represents a very unpredictable source of vitamin K. Second, there is some evidence that even small amounts of avocado can unpredictably alter the prothrombin time/INR.

16. Alcohol can alter the patient's response to COUMADIN® and thus increase or decrease the prothrombin time/INR. Alcohol should not be consumed by the patient on COUMADIN®.

17. The amount of vitamin K in leafy vegetables is highest in the outer, greener leaves when compared to the paler, inner leaves. The patient should take a balanced portion of the different leaves contained in the leafy vegetable. Also, the amount of vitamin K in iceberg lettuce is much lower than the amount of vitamin K in greener, more leafy types of lettuce.

How about eating SALADS? We suggest that the patient on COUMADIN® make salads out of iceberg lettuce only. Weigh the head of iceberg lettuce at the grocery store. At home, cut the lettuce into 8 to 10 equal portions (this is easy to do with a head of iceberg lettuce). Each portion of the head of lettuce will weigh about the same. Each ounce of iceberg lettuce contains about 9 micrograms of vitamin K. Simply multiply the number of ounces of lettuce you have in your salad by 9 (the number of micrograms of vitamin K per ounce of lettuce). The number you get is the number of micrograms of vitamin K in the portion of lettuce. For example, suppose your head of lettuce weighs 24 ounces. If you cut it into 8 equal portions, then each portion weighs 3 ounces. Each ounce contains 9 micrograms of vitamin K. Since 3 ounces times 9 micrograms per ounce equals 27 micrograms, there are 27 micrograms of vitamin K (approximately) in your portion of iceberg lettuce.

The effect of growing lettuce hydroponically is unknown and this type of lettuce should be avoided until more data is obtained in this regard. All data for lettuce available thus far is for lettuce grown the old-fashioned way.

18. Brewed black tea contains almost no vitamin K. Brewed green tea contains very little vitamin K. However, herbal teas should be avoided because they may contain herbs that may increase the effect of COUMADIN®.

LIST OF FOODS WITH VERY LOW VITAMIN K CONTENT

As stated previously, one of the purposes of this cookbook is to provide dietary guidelines so that the patient on COUMADIN® may consume approximately the same amount of vitamin K each day. To be successful, this cookbook must allow for a lot of different diets. Not everyone eats a big breakfast, for example. Towards this goal, this section contains a listing of foods with very little vitamin K content. With this list, patients on COUMADIN® can put into their diet any of the foods listed with little effect on their overall vitamin K intake. For example, if the patient prefers a small breakfast, he or she can enjoy a glass of cranberry juice, a cup of tea, and two pieces of toast without worrying about the vitamin K content. Similarly, of course, any other meal the patient wishes to make easily (from the standpoint of vitamin K calculation) could be made of a combination of the foods listed here. To take it one step further, this list also allows the easy addition of some food items to a meal that employs one or more of the recipes in the Recipe Section of the cookbook.

Please note that the criterion used to place a food on the following list was that it had to contain less than 2 micrograms (mcgs) of vitamin K per 100 grams (approximately 3 1/2 ounces) or milliliters.

- Apple juice
- Apple sauce
- Apple, skinless
- Bagel, plain
- Baking powder
- Banana
- Barley products (flour, bread)
- Beef
- Black olives
- Black pepper
- Bran flakes
- Bread (white, corn, or wheat)
- Cake (angel food)
- Chicken

- Coffee (caffeinated and decaffeinated)
- Cola
- Corn
- Corn flakes
- Corn oil
- Crackers (graham, wheat, or saltine, but watch out for additives, especially oils)
- Cranberry products (juice, sauce, etc.)
- Cream (Note: for every one per cent of fat in a milk product, there is only one-tenth of one microgram (mcg) of vitamin K per 100 grams or 100 milliliters)
- Cucumber, skinless
- Eel
- Egg white
- Egg yolk
- Eggplant
- Garlic and garlic powder
- Ginger ale
- Grapefruit, grapefruit juice
- Grapes, grape juice, grape jelly, etc.
- Honey
- Ice cream
- Jell-O
- Lemon juice, lemonade (the real stuff- not that artificial junk)
- Lemon peel
- Melon, cantaloupe
- Milk (see note above for "Cream")
- Millet
- Mushrooms
- Octopus
- Onions (but NOT spring onions)
- Oranges, orange juice
- Oysters
- Parsnips
- Peaches (canned)
- Peanuts (but NOT peanut butter)
- Pears (canned)
- Pineapple, pineapple juice

- Pork
- Pretzels
- Prunes, prune juice
- Radishes
- Raisins
- Rice, puffed rice, rice flour
- Sake
- Salmon
- Salt
- Sardine
- Shrimp
- Spaghetti
- Squid
- Sugar
- Tea, brewed (black only-not green)
- Tofu
- Turkey
- Turnips
- Vanilla
- Vinegar
- Wheat flour, wheat bread, puffed wheat, shredded wheat
- Wine
- Yellowtail (snapper)
- Yogurt, plain only

Some very common foods just missed making the list above. These include:
- Potato products which contain, when cooked, 10 micrograms of vitamin K per 100 grams,
- Tomato and tomato products (4 to 7 micrograms per 100 grams)
- Celery (12 micrograms per 100 grams)
- Cheddar cheese (3 micrograms per 100 grams)
- Oatmeal (3 micrograms per 100 grams)
- Peanut butter (10 micrograms per 100 grams)
- Squash (3 micrograms per 100 grams)

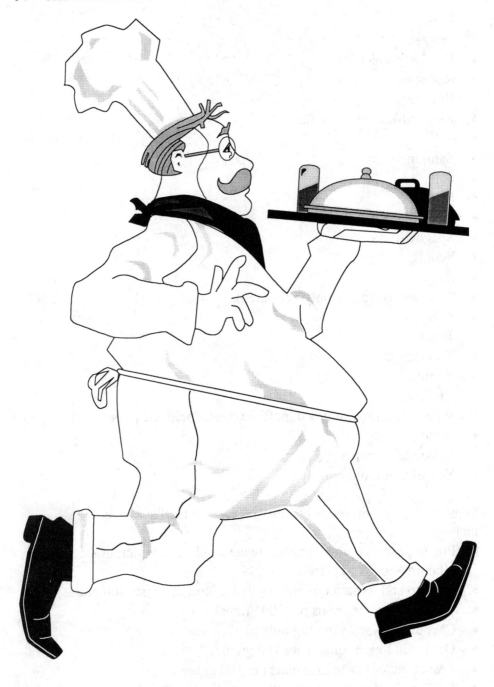

USEFUL INFORMATION FOR THE COOK

by GAIL BEYNON

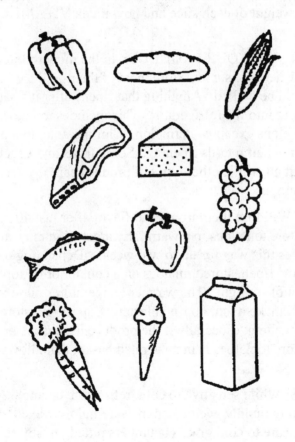

ODDS AND ENDS

HIGH ALTITUDE (3500 to 6500 feet) baking takes longer than at lower altitudes. Increase your baking time by about 1/4 to 1/3.

BREAD: When dealing with bread you need to make sure each slice you cut is approximately one ounce. (If you have a one pound loaf of bread and there are 16 slices then each slice is approximately one ounce.) When buying any uncut loaf of bread (Italian, French, etc.), note the weight of the loaf before cutting. That way you will be able to judge more accurately the weight of each slice and how much VITAMIN K you are getting.

DON'T CHILL ALL YOUR PRODUCE! In the modern kitchen, the refrigerator is where consumers store most of their produce. But not every food item should be chilled. Anything that ripens after it's harvested should not be put into the refrigerator. This includes tomatoes, unripe pears and all melons except watermelon. Chilling at temperatures below 55 degrees Fahrenheit retards ripening. Some fruits and vegetables should not be chilled at all, while other types of produce can be refrigerated with a few easy precautions.

TOMATOES: Will lose their aroma and flavor after just 40 minutes in the refrigerator. Store tomatoes in a warm, dry area. You may store vine-ripened tomatoes this way for up to two weeks. Depending on how fast you want them to ripen, store tomatoes on a counter or on top of the refrigerator, out of sunlight. The warmer temperatures on top of a refrigerator will make a tomato ripen faster. You should store tomatoes so that none are touching, especially if the produce has cracks or lesions. The best place to store tomatoes is in an aerated basket that allows plenty of air flow.

CUCUMBERS: While sensitive to cold, refrigerate cucumbers because they lose moisture rapidly even when they are lightly waxed. However, prolonged exposure to cold gives cucumbers pitted, mushy spots.

EGGPLANT: While sensitive to cold, refrigerate eggplant because they lose moisture rapidly. Store them in a paper bag in the refrigerator crisper drawer.

TROPICAL FRUITS: Never refrigerate any tropical fruit (such as bananas, mangos, papayas and others.) Only chill bananas if you do not want them to ripen any further. The skins will turn nearly black but the inside flesh can still be a normal white. You can freeze bananas before cooking. Just thaw and use as if they were fresh in baked goods. Frozen bananas cannot be used in gelatin desserts, banana splits, trifles, Banana Cream Pie, etc.

POTATOES AND SWEET POTATOES: When potatoes are refrigerated, their starch turns to sugar. While this condition can be reversed by removing the potatoes from the refrigerator, they will still retain some sugar, which causes them to brown when fried. Keep potatoes in a dark place slightly cooler than the normal temperature of the home, such as in a cool cupboard, in a basement storage area, or near the inside wall in a garage. In extremely cold conditions, covering the potatoes with a blanket or burlap will provide protection.

CITRUS FRUITS: For oranges, lemons, limes and grapefruit, refrigeration is a good way to preserve quality. Citrus fruits do not ripen further after harvest.

WINTER SQUASH OR MELONS: Refrigerate winter squash only after cooking, and refrigerate melons only after being cut open. These items maintain their best aroma and flavor at room temperature.

When storing produce, make liberal use of the crisper drawers. In most recently manufactured refrigerators, the crisper drawers can be somewhat adjusted for temperature and humidity. The crispers are usually marked 'fruits' or 'vegetables' or 'cool' and 'moist.' Store fruits and vegetables in paper or plastic bags with holes to slightly increase temperature and humidity.

Never store fruits and vegetables against the back wall of a refrigerator. The rear wall is the coldest area of any refrigerator and chilling injury or light freezing may occur.

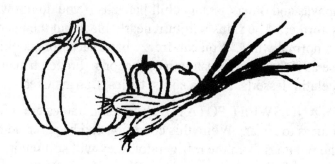

If produce becomes frozen, handle the produce carefully. When a celery or cabbage freezes, the cells are very sensitive to touch. Damage and bruising will occur unless they are allowed to thaw slowly with very little handling,

Do you have trouble digesting onions? Try using white onions rather than yellow onions. Some people are allergic to yellow onions but not white ones.

If you need to get walnut meats out whole, soak the nuts overnight in salt water before you crack them.

If the juice from your fresh fruit pie runs over in the oven, shake some salt on the spill. This causes the juice to burn to a crisp for easy removal.

Adding a little milk to the water the CAULIFLOWER is cooking in will help to keep it remain attractively white.

If your stew is over salted, try adding 1 teaspoon of vinegar and 1 teaspoon of sugar, and then reheat. Or add a few more potatoes.

To keep egg yolks from crumbling, when slicing hard-cooked eggs, wet your knife between each cut.

SUBSTITUTIONS

When you need an ingredient and you don't have it perhaps you can make a substitution

ALLSPICE - 1 teaspoon = 1/2 teaspoon cinnamon and 1/8 teaspoon ground cloves. (Unknown amount of vitamin K. Use sparingly.)

ARROWROOT - 2 teaspoon = 1 tablespoon cornstarch.

BAKING POWDER - 2 parts cream of tartar to 1 part baking soda. This will be a single-acting baking powder.

BREAD CRUMBS - 1/4 cup dry bread crumbs = 1 slice bread, 1/2 cup soft bread crumbs = 1 slice.

BUTTER - 1 cup butter = 7/8 cup oil OR 1 cup mayonnaise.

BUTTERMILK - Add 1 tablespoon lemon juice or white vinegar to 1 cup of milk and let stand for about 10 minutes or use 1 cup plain lowfat yogurt. Some grocery, health food and specialty stores carry buttermilk powder. Use it as you would any other dried milk powder.

CATSUP - 1/2 cup = 1/2 cup tomato sauce, 2 tablespoons sugar, 1 tablespoon vinegar, 1/8 teaspoon ground cloves.

CHOCOLATE - For 1 ounce of unsweetened chocolate use 3 tablespoons cocoa plus 1 tablespoon unsalted butter or Canola oil. For 1 2/3 ounces of sweetened chocolate use 1 ounce of unsweetened plus 4 teaspoon sugar.

COFFEE - 1/2 cup strong brewed coffee = 1 teaspoon instant coffee in 1/2 cup water.

CRACKER CRUMBS - 3/4 cup = 1 cup bread crumbs.

CREAM, COFFEE - 1 cup coffee cream = 3 tablespoons butter, plus about 3/4 cup milk

CREAM, LIGHT - 1 cup light cream = 7/8 cup milk plus 3 teaspoon butter.

CREAM, HEAVY - 1 cup heavy cream = 1/3 cup butter, plus about 3/4 cup milk (it will not whip!) OR 2/3 cup well-chilled evaporated milk, whipped OR 1 cup nonfat dry milk powder whipped with 1 cup ice water.

CREAM, SOUR - 1 cup = 3 tablespoon butter plus 7/8 cup buttermilk or yogurt. For dips, 1 cup = 1 cup cottage cheese pureed with 1/4 cup yogurt or buttermilk, or 6 ounce cream cheese plus enough milk to make 1 cup.

EGG YOLKS (for thickening) - 2 egg yolks = 1 whole egg.

FLOUR, PASTRY - Use 2 parts bread flour to 3 parts cake flour OR 5 parts all-purpose flour to 1 part cake flour.

FLOUR, ALL PURPOSE - To substitute cake flour for all-purpose flour: add 2 additional tablespoons for every cup called for in the recipe.

FLOUR, CAKE - Use 3 parts all-purpose flour to 1 part cornstarch.

FLOUR, SELF-RISING - use 1 1/4 teaspoons baking powder plus a pinch of salt for every cup of all-purpose flour.

FLOUR, THICKENING - 1 tablespoon flour for thickening: use 1 tablespoon quick cooking tapioca OR 1 1/2 teaspoon cornstarch, potato starch or arrowroot.

GARLIC - 1 clove = 1/2 teaspoon powdered, OR 1 teaspoon garlic salt (reduce added salt by 1/2 teaspoon).

GELATIN - A 1/4 ounce envelope = a little less than one tablespoon.

GINGER - 1 tablespoon fresh = 1 teaspoon powdered or 1 tablespoon candied with sugar washed off.

HERBS - 1 tablespoon fresh = 1 teaspoon dried (Dried herbs are very high in VITAMIN K).

HONEY - For 1 cup: use 1 1/4 cup sugar plus 1/3 cup liquid. For baking, also decrease the liquid in the recipe by 1/4 cup. If there is no liquid in the recipe, add an additional 1/4 cup flour. Unless sour cream or sour milk is used in the recipe, add a pinch of baking soda.

HOT PEPPER SAUCE - Few drops = dash of cayenne or red pepper.

LEMON JUICE - 1 teaspoon = 1/2 teaspoon vinegar. Juice of 1 lemon is about 2-3 tablespoons of lemon juice.

LIME JUICE - Use equivalent amount of lemon juice. Juice of 1 lime is about 2 tablespoons lime juice.

MILK, FRESH SWEET MILK: 1/2 cup evaporated milk plus 1/2 cup water OR 1/4 cup dried skim milk powder plus 1 cup water and 2 teaspoon melted butter or oil OR 1 cup skim milk plus 2 teaspoon melted butter or oil.

MILK, SOUR - 1 cup sour milk = 1 cup sweet milk plus 1 tablespoon vinegar or lemon juice

MILK, SKIM - 1/3 cup instant powdered milk plus 3/4 cup water. In baking: 1 cup whole milk = 1 cup fruit juice.

MILK, SWEETENED CONDENSED - 1 cup milk plus 2 tablespoons of nonfat powdered milk, 1/2 cup boiling water and 3/4 cup sugar. Beat for 10 minutes. Then chill. Use as a substitute for sweetened condensed milk.

MUSHROOMS - 6 ounces of canned drained mushrooms = 1/2 pound mushrooms.

MUSTARD - 1 tablespoon prepared = 1 teaspoon dried.

OIL - In cakes you can usually replace 1/2 the oil with an equal amount of applesauce. Mayonnaise can be substituted for an equal amount of oil in most baked dishes.

OLIVE OIL - Use a good quality oil for the best flavor. If you do not use a lot of oil you should buy small quantities at a time. Oil will go rancid.

ONION - 1 small fresh chopped onion = 1 tablespoon dried minced or 1/4 cup frozen chopped onion.

ORANGE JUICE - Juice of 1 orange is about 1/3 to 1/2 cup orange juice.

RAISINS - 1/2 cup = 1/2 cup cut up pitted prunes or dates.

SALT - When making a brine, do not use low sodium salt. Low sodium salt as a flavor enhancer is fine.

SOY SAUCE - 1/4 cup = 3 tablespoons of Worcestershire sauce plus 1 tablespoon water.

SUGAR, BROWN - Use 1 to 2 tablespoons molasses to 1 cup of granulated sugar OR substitute 1 cup granulated for 1 cup firmly packed brown sugar.

SUGAR, GRANULATED - To use honey, combine 3/4 cup honey, plus 1 tablespoon honey, plus a pinch of baking soda for every 1 cup of sugar. Reduce the liquid in the recipe by 3 tablespoons. Do not replace more than 1/3 of the sugar with honey. If using molasses, combine 1 cup molasses plus 1/2 teaspoon baking soda for every 1 cup sugar and reduce the liquid in the recipe by 4 teaspoons. Do not replace more than 1/2 of the sugar with the molasses. One cup sugar = 1 3/4 cups confectioner's sugar but do not substitute in baking.

SUGAR, TURBINADO - 1 cup = 1 cup granulated with a heavier molasses flavor.

TOMATO JUICE - Three cups = 1 1/2 cup tomato sauce plus 1 1/2 cup water OR one (6 ounce) can of tomato paste plus 3 cans of water and a dash of salt and pepper.

TOMATO PASTE - 1 tablespoon = 1 tablespoon catsup.

TOMATO PUREE - 1 cup puree = 1/2 cup paste plus 1/2 cup water.

TOMATO SAUCE - 1 cup tomato sauce = 1 can tomato paste plus 1 1/2 cans of water.

TOMATOES - 1 cup canned = 1 1/3 cup chopped fresh tomatoes simmered.

WINE FOR MARINADE - 1/2 cup wine = 1/4 cup vinegar plus 1 tablespoon sugar plus 1/4 cup water.

WORCESTERSHIRE SAUCE - 1 teaspoon Worcestershire sauce = 1 tablespoon soy sauce plus a dash of hot pepper sauce.

YEAST - 1 cake compressed yeast = 1 package dried, 1 package dried = 1 scant tablespoon.

YOGURT - 1 cup yogurt = 1 cup buttermilk.

ONE OUNCE (30 GRAMS) FOOD MEASURES

2	tablespoons	Butter
1	square	Bitter chocolate
4	tablespoons	Flour
2 1/2	cups	Dried hops
2	tablespoons	Liquid
1	tablespoon	Salt
2	tablespoons	Soda
2	tablespoons	Sugar

MEASUREMENT CHART

1 tablespoon	=	3 teaspoons
3/4 tablespoon	=	2 1/4 teaspoons
1/2 tablespoon	=	1 1/2 teaspoons
1/3 tablespoon	=	1 teaspoon
Pinch	=	Less than 1/8 teaspoon
1 cup	=	16 tablespoons
1/2 cup	=	8 tablespoons
1/3 cup	=	5 1/3 tablespoons
1/4 cup	=	4 tablespoons
1 gallon	=	4 quarts or 8 pints or 16 cups
1 quart	=	2 pints or 4 cups
1 pint	=	2 cups
1 pound	=	16 ounces
3/4 pound	=	12 ounces
2/3 pound	=	10 2/3 ounces
1/2 pound	=	8 ounces
1/3 pound	=	5 1/3 ounces
1/4 pound	=	4 ounces

ONE POUND (450 GRAMS) FOOD MEASURES

(16 ounces (dry) per pound, 4 ounces per 1/4 pound)

2 1/2	cups	Shelled almonds
2 1/2	cups	Dry beans
2	cups	Butter
2 2/3	cups	Dried currants
2 1/2	cups	Pitted dates
9-10		Eggs, with shells
3 3/4	cups	Whole-wheat flour
4	cups	White flour
3 3/4	cups	Rye flour
2	cups	Liquid
3	cups	Cornmeal
2	cups	Chopped meats
2	cups	Milk
4	cups	Shelled nuts (about)
2 2/3	cups	Oatmeal
2	cups	Diced potatoes
2	good-sized	Whole potatoes
2 2/3	cups	Seedless raisins
2 1/2	cups	Long-grain rice
2	cups	Granulated sugar
2 1/4	cups	Brown sugar
3 1/2	cups	Powdered sugar
3 2/3	cups	Shelled walnuts
4	cups	Crumbs
3	cups	Candied fruit
5	cups	Coffee (ground)

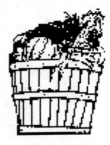

APPETIZERS

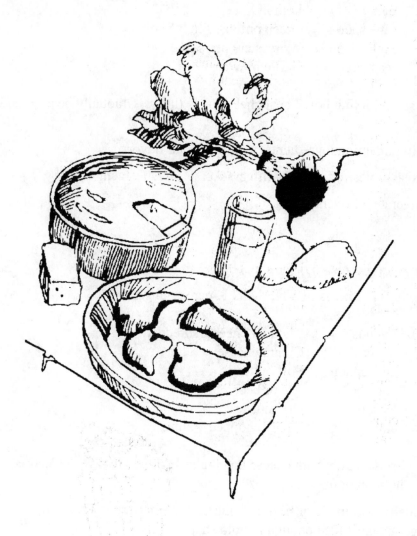

SHRIMP SPREAD

2 servings (7 mcgs of VITAMIN K per serving.)

16	ounces	Cream cheese, softened
1/2	pound	Shrimp, cooked, chopped
1	tablespoon	Prepared horseradish
1/4	teaspoon	Pepper
1/4	cup	Lemon juice
1	tablespoon	Green onions, finely chop
1	tablespoon	Worcestershire sauce
1/8	teaspoon	Garlic powder

In a small mixing bowl, beat cheese until fluffy. Gradually beat in lemon juice.

Stir in remaining ingredients. Chill to blend flavors.

Garnish as desired. Serve with crackers or fresh vegetables.

Refrigerate leftovers.

CHEDDAR-ALE CHEESE LOGS

8 servings (12 mcgs of VITAMIN K per serving.)

1 1/2	pounds	Cheddar cheese, shredded
3	ounces	Cream cheese
4	tablespoons	Soft butter
3/4	cup	Ale or beer
1	teaspoon	Dry mustard
1/2	cup	Finely chopped walnuts

Beat cheddar and cream cheese and butter in large bowl with electric mixer until smooth.

Gradually beat in ale or beer and mustard. If mixture is very soft, refrigerate until firm enough to hold shape.

Divide mixture in half and shape into two logs. Press a 3 inch round of wax paper onto the end of each log to keep area free from walnuts.

Put walnuts and on a sheet of wax paper.

Roll cheese logs in nut mixture to cover completely. Place on serving plates or boards, remove paper rounds.

Decorate with pimiento.

To keep, cover with plastic wrap and refrigerate. Keeps well for several weeks. Do not roll in nuts or decorate until ready to use.

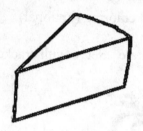

AMARETTO CHEESE SPREAD

12 servings (8 mcgs of VITAMIN K per serving.)

16	ounces	Cream cheese, softened
8	ounces	Pineapple, crushed, drained
1/2	cup	Green pepper, chopped fine
3	tablespoons	Green onions, chopped
3	tablespoons	Amaretto
1	teaspoon	Seasoned salt
1	cup	Almond slivers, chopped, toasted

Mix first six ingredients and half of the almonds.

Form mixture into a ball. Roll in the remaining almonds. Refrigerate several hours. Serve with crackers.

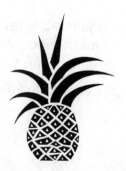

DRIED TOMATO SMOKY SPREAD
12 servings (5 mcgs of VITAMIN K per serving.)

16	ounces	Cream cheese, softened
1	teaspoon	Liquid Smoke
6	tomatoes	Dried, no oil
		Orange food coloring (optional)

Mix all in food processor. Refrigerate. Serve with crackers.

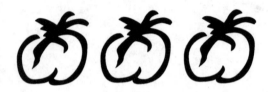

STUFFED MUSHROOMS
6 servings (3 mcgs of VITAMIN K per serving.)

12	ounces	Large mushrooms
1/4	pound	Butter
1	tablespoon	Olive oil, treated (See DIETARY TIP # 10.)
1/4	teaspoon	Garlic powder
2	tablespoons	White wine
1/4	teaspoon	Fresh basil, minced
1/4	teaspoon	Fresh oregano, minced
1	cup	Bread crumbs
1/2	cup	Grated cheddar or Swiss cheese

Wash mushrooms and remove stems. Put the caps on baking sheet. Brown stems in butter. Mix the stems and all of the rest of the ingredients together. Stuff the caps.

Bake for 15 to 20 minutes until brown. (Shrimp added to this is good.)

VERMONT CHEDDAR AND MAPLE CRACKERS

8 servings (4 mcgs of VITAMIN K per serving.)

2	cups	Shredded sharp cheddar
2 1/2	ounces	Chopped pecan pieces
1/3	cup	Mayonnaise, homemade (See Recipe Index.)
1	tablespoon	Maple syrup
1/2	teaspoon	Worcestershire sauce
36		Whole-grain crackers

Mix the cheese, pecans, mayonnaise, maple syrup and Worcestershire sauce together in a medium-sized bowl. Spread the mixture by rounded teaspoonfuls evenly on the crackers.

Place the crackers on a flat pan or cookie sheet and run it under the broiler until the cheese is melted and bubbling. Transfer the crackers to a plate and serve at once. Makes 3 dozen puffs.

MIXED ANTIPASTO PLATTER

8 servings (11 mcgs of VITAMIN K per serving.)

2	cloves	Garlic
24	slices	Hard-crusted Italian bread, each 1/2-inch thick
12	slices	Prosciutto or fully cooked Virginia ham, cut in half
12	slices	Provolone cheese, cut in half
24	slices	Genoa salami
24		Marinated mushrooms
24		Marinated artichoke hearts
24		Pickled imported Italian black olives, pitted
1/2	cup	Extra-virgin olive oil, treated (See DIETARY TIP # 10.)
		Juice of 1/2 lemon
1	teaspoon	Fresh oregano

Cut each clove garlic in half and rub cut sides over both sides of bread. Arrange bread in single layer on serving platter.

Top each bread slice with prosciutto, cheese, salami, mushrooms, artichoke hearts and olives. Drizzle with oil. Squeeze lemon juice over top and sprinkle with oregano.

CRACKERS DEL PASEO

10 servings (8 mcgs of VITAMIN K per serving.)

1	cup	Mayonnaise, homemade (See Recipe Index.)
3/4	cup	Cheddar cheese, grated
1/2	teaspoon	Dry mustard
1/2	teaspoon	Caraway seeds
1	medium	Onion, thinly sliced
50		Butter crackers
		Additional mayonnaise for crackers

Mix mayonnaise, cheese, mustard and caraway seeds.

Spread Ritz crackers with a thin layer of mayonnaise and top with a slice of onion.

Add a teaspoonful of the mixture on top of onion. Place under broiler until hot.

Serve immediately.

GARLICKY CLAM DIP

8 servings (Less than 1 mcg of VITAMIN K per serving.)

8	ounces	Cream cheese
1/2	teaspoon	Salt
1/2	tablespoon	Garlic
		Fresh ground pepper (dash)
7	ounces	Clams, drained and minced
1/4	cup	Clam broth
1 1/2	teaspoon	Worcestershire
2	teaspoons	Lemon juice

Using garlic press, squeeze pulp and juice into softened cheese. Cream with a spoon until smooth. Gradually add the remaining ingredients, blending until smooth.

For thinner dip, add more clam broth.

Serve with crackers, chips or veggies.

CRAB DIP

8 servings (12 mcgs of VITAMIN K per serving.)

1	pound	Crab meat
1/2	cup	Mayonnaise, homemade (See Recipe Index.)
		Garlic salt, to taste
2	tablespoons	Onion, grated
2	teaspoons	Prepared mustard
2	teaspoons	Powdered sugar
2/3	cup	White wine

Mix together all ingredients except crab meat. Heat slowly. Add Crab meat. Serve warm with crackers.

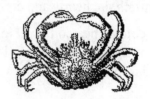

TANGY BLUE CHEESE DIP

4 servings (3 mcgs of VITAMIN K per serving.)

1/2	cup	Blue cheese, crumbled
1 1/2	cups	Sour cream
1	teaspoon	Garlic, minced
2	tablespoons	Fresh chives, finely chopped
1/8	teaspoon	Hot sauce

Blend the blue cheese and sour cream thoroughly.

Add all the other ingredients, blending well. Cover and chill. Makes about 2 cups of dip.

SUGGESTED DIPPERS: Carrots, Cherry Tomatoes, Pineapple, Asian Pear, Cocktail Black Bread, Italian Or French Bread Chunks.

ARTICHOKE DIP

4 servings (19 mcgs of VITAMIN K per serving.)

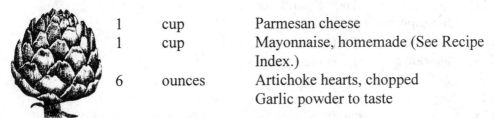

1	cup	Parmesan cheese
1	cup	Mayonnaise, homemade (See Recipe Index.)
6	ounces	Artichoke hearts, chopped
		Garlic powder to taste

Combine equal amounts Parmesan cheese and mayonnaise. Add garlic powder. Add artichoke hearts and combine.

May be served cold or heated for 10 to 20 minutes in a 350 degree Fahrenheit oven until cheese melts. (Do not heat in microwave.) Serve with chips or as a spread on French bread.

GOLDEN CITRUS-RAISIN DIP

6 servings (5 mcgs of VITAMIN K per serving.)

1	medium	Orange, peeled, seeded and quartered
1	cup	Pecans, chopped
2	cups	Golden raisins
1/2	cup	Mayonnaise, homemade (See Recipe Index.)
1/2	cup	Plain yogurt

Combine all of the ingredients in a food processor or blender and process to a chunky consistency. Cover and chill. Makes about 4 1/2 cups of dip.

SUGGESTED DIPPERS: Ladyfingers, Plum Wafers, Pineapple, Ham, Chicken Drumettes, Celery.

CAESAR MAYO DIP

6 servings (15 mcgs of VITAMIN K per serving.)

2		Anchovy fillets
1 1/2	cups	Mayonnaise, homemade (See Recipe Index.)
1	teaspoon	Dijon mustard
2	tablespoons	Parmesan cheese
1	teaspoon	Worcestershire sauce
1	tablespoon	Lemon juice
1/4	teaspoon	Black pepper

Chop and mash the anchovy fillets on a cutting board. Put in a bowl and blend in the mayonnaise. Add the remaining ingredients and blend well. Cover and chill. Makes about 1 3/4 cups of dip.

SUGGESTED DIPPERS: Shrimp, Deli Roast Beef, Turkey or Radishes.

TIPSY TUNA DIP

12 servings (8 mcgs of VITAMIN K per serving.)

1 1/2	tablespoons	Brandy
1	cup	Cream cheese, softened
1/4	cup	Sour cream
1/4	cup	Mayonnaise, homemade (See Recipe Index.)
3/4	cup	Fresh tuna, flaked, or
6 1/2	ounces	Tuna, flaked, water pack, well drained
2	tablespoons	Onion, minced
1	tablespoon	Lemon juice
1/8	teaspoon	Hot sauce
1/8	teaspoon	Salt

Beat the brandy and cream cheese to a smooth and creamy consistency. Blend in the sour cream and mayonnaise. Mix in the tuna and onion, blending well. Add the remaining ingredients and blend until almost smooth. May be served at room temperature or chilled. Makes about 2 1/2 cups of dip.

SUGGESTED DIPPERS: French Bread Cubes, Cheese Crackers, Bread Sticks, Carrots & Radishes.

CAPONATA (EGGPLANT APPETIZER)

8 servings (11 mcgs of VITAMIN K per serving.)

1/4	cup	Oil, olive or Canola, treated (See DIETARY TIP # 10.)
1	small	Eggplant, peeled, cut in 1 inch cubes
1 1/2	cups	Celery, cut in 1/2-inch slices
1/2	cup	Pitted black olives, chopped
1	cup	Onion, minced
1	clove	Garlic, crushed
1/4	teaspoon	Fresh dill
3/4	cup	Tomato puree
1/2	cup	Water
1/4	cup	Vinegar
1	tablespoon	Sugar
1	teaspoon	Salt

Heat oil in large skillet and fry eggplant cubes until lightly browned. Add celery, olives, onion and garlic. Cook until vegetables are crisp tender.

Combine tomato paste, water, vinegar, sugar and salt. Pour over vegetables in skillet, stir lightly and simmer 1 minute. Remove from heat. Cool and place in covered container in refrigerator until thoroughly chilled. Serve.

Makes 3 to 4 cups.

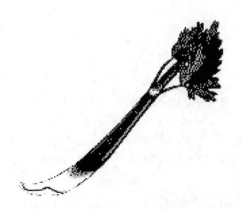

CRAB-MELT CANAPÉS

8 servings (3 mcgs of VITAMIN K per serving.)

8	ounces	Crab meat (about 1 cup)
1/4	pound	Jarlsberg or Swiss cheese, shredded
1/4	cup	Mayonnaise, homemade (See Recipe Index.)
1/4	teaspoon	Dry mustard
30		Melba toast rounds
1/2	cup	Sliced pitted black ripe olives
3/4	teaspoon	Black pepper, coarsely ground

About 30 minutes before serving or early in the day, chop crab meat. In a small bowl, with a fork, mix crab meat, cheese, mayonnaise, dry mustard, and 1/4 teaspoon coarsely ground black pepper. Spread 1 heaping teaspoon of the crab meat mixture on each melba toast round. Place on cookie sheets, sprinkle with 1/2 teaspoon coarsely ground black pepper.

If not serving right away, cover and refrigerate. About 15 minutes before serving: preheat broiler. Broil canapés about 3 minutes or until cheese melts. Top each canapé with a slice of ripe olive.

Arrange canapés and garnish on platter. Serve immediately. Makes 2 1/2 dozen canapés.

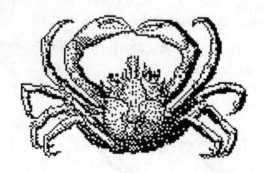

SALMON AND GOUDA PATE

15 servings (10 mcgs of VITAMIN K per serving.)

7	ounces	Gouda, smoked, shredded
3	ounces	Cream cheese cubed
3	tablespoons	Milk
1/4	cup	Butter
1/3	cup	Mayonnaise, homemade (See Recipe Index.)
1/4	cup	Green onion, finely chopped
2	tablespoons	Lemon juice
1/4	teaspoon	Garlic salt
1/8	teaspoon	Hot pepper sauce
1	pound	Salmon, cooked or 14 ounce canned salmon
1/3	cup	Almonds toasted
		Lemon slices
		Breads and crackers

Mix gouda, cream cheese and milk. Set aside.

Beat butter until fluffy. Beat in mayonnaise, green onion, lemon juice, garlic salt and hot pepper sauce. Add salmon, beat until combined.

Line bottom and sides of 8 x 4 x 2 inch loaf pan with plastic wrap. Sprinkle almonds in bottom of pan. Carefully spoon in half of the salmon mixture and spread evenly. Spread cheese mixture on top of salmon layer. Spread with remaining salmon mixture. Cover and chill for 6 to 24 hours.

Turn out onto serving plate and carefully peel off the plastic wrap. Serve with crackers and/or bread.

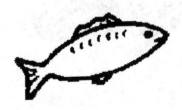

DEVILED EGGS

12 servings (Less than 1 mcg of VITAMIN K per serving.)

6		Warm hard-cooked eggs
1/4	cup	Plain yogurt
1/4	teaspoon	Salt
1/2	teaspoon	Worcestershire
1/4	teaspoon	Dry mustard
1	teaspoon	Lemon juice
		Paprika

Slice eggs in half lengthwise, remove yolks and mash them. Add remaining ingredients except paprika. Mix until smooth. Fill egg whites with mixture, chill. Dust with paprika and serve.

CANTALOUPE FRUIT SALAD

6 servings (11 mcgs of VITAMIN K per serving.)

2	medium	Cantaloupes, peeled and seeded
1	large	Pineapple, cored, peeled and cut in chunks
1	cup	Raisins
1	cup	Finely chopped walnuts
1	large	Apple, peeled, cored and cut in small chunks
		Vanilla fat-free yogurt

Cut the cantaloupes into small chunks and mix with all the other fruits and the walnuts in a large salad bowl. Scoop yogurt into individual serving bowls and pass the fruit salad. Stir to coat and eat.

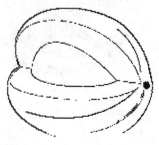

SALMON MOUSSE

12 servings (2 mcgs of VITAMIN K per serving.)

1	envelope	Unflavored gelatin
1/4	cup	Cold dry white wine or water
1/2	cup	Boiling water
1/4	cup	Sour cream
1/4	cup	Mayonnaise, homemade (See Recipe Index.)
1	tablespoon	Fresh lemon juice
1	teaspoon	Salt
1/8	teaspoon	Hot pepper sauce
1	tablespoon	Minced onion
1/4	teaspoon	Paprika
5	ounces	Canned salmon, skin and bones removed, flaked
1	cup	Heavy cream

In a large heat proof bowl, soften gelatin in cold wine. Slowly stir in boiling water until gelatin dissolves. Let cool to room temperature. Whisk in mayonnaise, sour cream, lemon juice, onion, salt, paprika, and hot sauce until well blended. Refrigerate until mixture begins to thicken, about 20 minutes. Mix in salmon.

In another large bowl, whip cream until soft peaks form. Fold whipped cream into salmon mixture, one-third at a time, until well blended. Pour mixture into an oiled 5- or 6-cup mold. Cover and refrigerate until firm, at least 4 hours or as long as 2 days. Unmold onto a serving plate and serve chilled.

COMMENTS: Serve this mild mousse with dark pumpernickel bread and peeled cucumber slices.

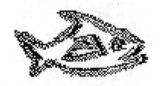

CARAMELIZED CARNITAS

10 servings (Less than 1 mcg of VITAMIN K per serving.)

1 1/2	pounds	Pork shoulder, boneless
2	tablespoons	Brown sugar, packed
1	tablespoon	Tequila
1	tablespoon	Molasses
1/2	teaspoon	Salt
1/4	teaspoon	Pepper
2	cloves	Garlic, finely chopped
1/3	cup	Water
1		Green onion with top, sliced for garnish

Cut pork into 1-inch cubes. Place pork cubes in single layer in 10-inch skillet. Top with remaining ingredients except green onion.

Heat to boiling, reduce heat. Simmer uncovered, stirring occasionally, until the water has evaporated and the pork is slightly caramelized, about 35 minutes.

Sprinkle with green onion and serve with wooden picks.

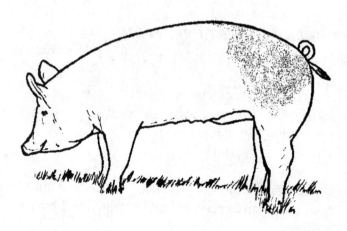

GRILLED BRUSCHETTA WITH FRESH MOZZARELLA AND TOMATOES

12 servings (5 mcgs of VITAMIN K per serving.)

12		1 1/2 inch slices sourdough or Italian bread
1/2	cup	Extra virgin olive oil, treated (See DIETARY TIP # 10.)
1	cup	Tomato, finely diced
2	cloves	Garlic crushed
12	slices	Fresh mozzarella (No more than 1 ounce per slice)
12		Whole fresh basil leaves

Rub bread with garlic and drizzle olive oil over it. Grill slices over an open flame, turning once until crisp. Top with mozzarella and place in 375 degree Fahrenheit oven until cheese just begins to melt. Remove to serving plates. Garnish with tomato and basil leaves (one basil leaf per bruschetta).

BLACK CHERRY YOGURT CREAM DIP

6 servings (1 mcg of VITAMIN K per serving.)

8	ounces	Black cherry yogurt
3	ounces	Cream cheese, softened
1	tablespoon	Powdered sugar
1/4	teaspoon	Vanilla

In a blender, combine all the ingredients. Process 1-2 minutes or until smooth. Pour into a small serving bowl, refrigerate 2 hours or until slightly thickened.

Serve with fresh fruit dippers. (Change the dip flavor by changing the type of fruit yogurt.)

EGGPLANT CAVIAR

10 servings (6 mcgs of VITAMIN K per serving.)

3	cups	Eggplant, peeled and 1/2 inch cubes
1/3	cup	Chopped green pepper
1		Medium white onion, minced
3		Cloves garlic
1/3	cup	Oil, olive or Canola, treated (See DIETARY TIP # 10.)
6	ounces	Tomato paste
4	ounces	Canned mushroom stems and pieces, undrained
1/2	cup	Pimento stuffed olives
1/4	cup	Water
2	tablespoons	Red wine vinegar
1 1/2	teaspoon	Sugar
1	teaspoon	Seasoned salt
1/2	teaspoon	Oregano, fresh minced
1/4	teaspoon	Pepper

Put eggplant, green pepper, garlic and oil in skillet. Cover and cook gently for about 10 minutes, stirring occasionally.

Add tomato paste, mushrooms (with liquid) and remaining ingredients.

Cover and simmer 45 minutes to an hour to get a thick consistency. Turn into covered dish and refrigerate overnight to blend flavors.

Serve with crackers and chips. Makes about 1 quart and freezes well. To make this lower in fat, reduce the oil to 1 tablespoon. I have also left out the onion and it tastes great that way too.

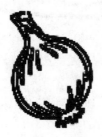

CROSTINI A LA PORCINI

8 servings (2 mcgs of VITAMIN K per serving.)

1	clove	Garlic, minced
1	ounces	Imported dried porcini mushrooms
3	tablespoons	Olive oil, treated (See DIETARY TIP # 10.)
1	tablespoon	Unsalted butter
1/2	pound	Fresh shiitake or chanterelle mushrooms, sliced (or white button, or a mixture)
1/4	cup	Heavy cream
3	tablespoons	Fresh grated Asiago or Parmesan cheese
8	large	(Or 16 small) Slices Italian bread, lightly toasted

Soak porcini in 1 cup very hot water for 20 minutes. Drain and dice, removing any hard stem pieces. (Strain and save the liquid to use in soup.)

Heat oil and butter in a large skillet until butter foams. Add mushrooms and cook until lightly golden. Add garlic and cook and stir for one minute. Add cream and cook until slightly thickened, about 5 minutes.

Season to taste with salt and a couple of grinds of black pepper. Cool slightly (can be made ahead) and mound on toast. Sprinkle with cheese and run under a preheated broiler until cheese is melted and all is bubbly and beginning to brown. Serve immediately.

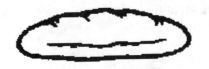

BREADS, SANDWICHES & SPREADS

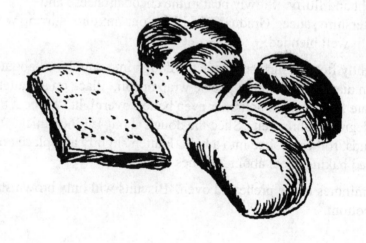

CHEDDAR BISCUITS

8 servings (VITAMIN K content = 6 mcg per serving)

2	cups	Unbleached flour
1	teaspoon	Mustard, dry
1	teaspoon	Paprika
1/4	teaspoon	Baking powder
1	cup	Butter, room temperature
10	ounces	Cheddar, sharp, grated
1	teaspoon	Worcestershire Sauce

Combine the flour, dry mustard, paprika and baking powder in a medium bowl.

Beat the butter (either by hand or with an electric mixer at medium speed) until light and fluffy. Slowly beat in the cheddar cheese and Worcestershire sauce. Gradually add the flour mixture, stirring with a fork, until well blended.

On a lightly floured surface, shape the dough into a long roll about 1 3/4-inches in diameter. Wrap in plastic wrap or foil. Place on a platter and refrigerate for at least 2 hours, or even better, overnight. Preheat the oven to 325 degrees Fahrenheit. Slice the dough about 1/3 inch thick. With your hands, roll each slice into a ball. Flatten slightly and place on an ungreased baking sheet about 2 inches apart.

Bake 8 minutes in the preheated oven. Biscuits will only brown slightly on the bottom.

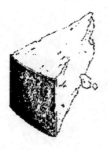

GARDEN PIZZA

8 Servings (25 mcgs of VITAMIN K per serving.)

1	12 inch	PIZZA DOUGH CRUST (See Recipe Index)
2	cups	Mushrooms, sliced
1 1/2	cups	Carrot, shredded
1	cup	Zucchini, peeled and finely sliced
1/2	cup	Onion, chopped
1	tablespoon	Canola or olive oil, treated (See DIETARY TIP # 10.)
8	ounces	Tomato sauce
1/2	teaspoon	Garlic
1/2	teaspoon	Fennel seed
1	teaspoon	Fresh basil
1	teaspoon	Fresh oregano
1	teaspoon	Brown sugar
1	cup	Mozzarella cheese
1/2	cup	Parmesan cheese

Pre-heat oven to 425 degrees Fahrenheit and put your prepared crust onto a pizza pan and bake for 14 to 16 minutes.

Meanwhile, sauté mushrooms, carrots, zucchini and onion in oil over medium heat for 3 minutes.

When crust is prebaked, sprinkle with vegetables, sauce, seasonings, sugar and cheeses. Bake for 20 minutes.

Remove from oven and cool for 3 minutes before serving.

  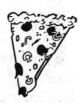

PIZZA DOUGH:

8 servings (VITAMIN K content = 1 mcg per serving)

1	packet	Fresh or dry yeast (1 scant tablespoon)
1/4	cup	Warm water
1	tablespoon	Honey
3	tablespoons	Olive oil, treated (See DIETARY TIP # 10.)
3/4	cup	Cool water
3	cups	All purpose flour

Dissolve yeast in the 1/4 cup warm water and let proof for 10 minutes. Meanwhile, combine the salt, honey, olive oil and cool water in a small bowl and mix well.

Place the flour in a large bowl and make a well in the center. Pour the honey-water mixture and proofed yeast into the well. Slowly incorporate the flour into the wet ingredients. When the dough is formed, transfer it to a lightly floured surface and knead until smooth. (You can knead this in a mixer equipped with a dough hook.). Place in a buttered bowl and let rest, covered, for 30 minutes. Divide the dough into 4 equal parts (or leave as one to make one very large pizza).

Form each part into smooth, tight balls. Place on a flat dish, cover with a damp towel and refrigerate at least 2 hours.

One hour before baking, remove the dough from the refrigerator. If you use a pizza pan, grease it well and flatten the dough out and spread in the pizza pan making the outer edge thicker for the rim. At this point you can let the dough rise again for half an hour if you like a lighter dough (although you do not need to).

Bake the dough at 350 degrees Fahrenheit for 10 to 12 minutes. Remove from oven. At this point you have a pizza dough crust to use for any type pizza.

Cover with sauce and your favorite toppings. Bake at 500 degrees Fahrenheit for 10 to 12 minutes. If you have a baking stone, let the stone heat in a 500 degree Fahrenheit oven for at least 30 minutes to an hour before putting in the pizza. (Don't forget to add the vitamin K content of the foods you use to top the pizza.)

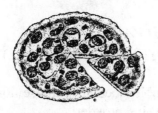

CHEDDAR FANS

12 fans (2 mcgs of VITAMIN K per serving.)

5	ounces	Cheddar, sharp, grated
2	cups	Unbleached flour, sifted
1	tablespoon	Baking powder
1	teaspoon	Salt
1/2	cup	Butter
1/2	cup	Milk
1/2	cup	Butter, softened
1/4	cup	Butter, melted

Grease the bottoms of 12 muffin pan cups. Grate the cheese into a bowl, if not already grated and set aside.

Sift the flour, baking powder and salt into a bowl. Cut in the butter with a pastry blender or two knives, until the mixture resembles coarse corn meal.

Make a well in the center of the mixture and add the milk all at once. Stir with a fork until the dough forms a ball. Gently form the dough into a ball and put on a lightly floured surface. Knead it lightly with the fingertips 10 or 15 times.

Roll the dough into a 12 by 10-inch rectangle about 1/4-inch thick. Cut into 5 strips and spread with the softened butter. Sprinkle four strips with the grated cheddar cheese and stack the four on top of one another and top with the fifth strip.

Cut into 12 equal pieces and place on end in the muffin cups. Brush the tops of the rolls with the melted butter. Bake at 450 degrees Fahrenheit for 10 to 15 minutes or until the biscuits are golden brown.

Serve hot with butter.

MUFFINS: BASIC AND VARIATIONS
12 servings (2 mcgs of VITAMIN K per serving.)

2	cups	Unbleached all-purpose flour
1	tablespoon	Baking powder
2	tablespoons	Granulated sugar
1	teaspoon	Salt
1	Large	Egg
1	cup	Milk
1/2	cup	Canola oil, treated (See DIETARY TIP # 10.)

Grease 12, 2 1/2-inch muffin cups. Heat oven to 400 degrees Fahrenheit.
Sift Flour, baking powder, sugar and salt into a medium-sized bowl. Stir
to mix well.

In a small bowl, beat egg with a fork. Add milk and oil. Add all at once
to dry ingredients. Stir mixture only until dry ingredients are moistened.

Batter will be lumpy. Drop batter from a tablespoon into prepared muffins
pans, filling each cup half to two-thirds full. Bake 15 to 20 minutes, or
until golden brown. Remove from pan and serve hot with butter, jam or
marmalade.

VARIATIONS:

GINGER MUFFINS:
Add 1/2 cup finely diced candied ginger to flour mixture before adding
liquid. (VITAMIN K per muffin = 2 mcg.)

BANANA PECAN MUFFINS:
Prepare muffin batter but use only 1/2 cup milk. Add 1/2 cup chopped
pecans and 1/4 teaspoon ground nutmeg to sifted flour. Add 1 cup
mashed, peeled banana with the egg, milk and oil. (VITAMIN K per
muffin = 4 mcg.)

BLUEBERRY MUFFINS:
Toss 1 cup washed and well-drained fresh or frozen blueberries with sifted
flour mixture before adding liquid. (VITAMIN K per muffin = 3 to 4
mcg.)

ORANGE MUFFINS:

Cut 2 peeled navel oranges into sections. When batter is in the cups, place an orange section on top of each and sprinkle lightly with granulated sugar. (VITAMIN K per muffin = 2 mcg.)

CHEESE MUFFINS:

Fold 1/2 cup grated sharp yellow cheese into muffin mix with the last few strokes of batter. Serve hot with scrambled eggs and bacon for a special breakfast. (VITAMIN K per muffin = 3 mcg.)

SURPRISE MUFFINS:

Fill muffin cups 1/3 full of batter. Drop 1/2 teaspoon of your favorite jelly in center of batter. Add batter to fill cup 2/3 full. Kids just love these as will you. (VITAMIN K per muffin = 2 mcg.)

BUTTERMILK BISCUITS

1 dozen (VITAMIN K content = 1 mcg per biscuit)

3	tablespoons	Canola oil, treated (See DIETARY TIP # 10.)
2/3	cup	Buttermilk, 1 % fat
2	cups	Flour
2	teaspoons	Baking powder
1/4	teaspoon	Baking soda
1/4	teaspoon	Salt
2	tablespoons	Sugar

Mix buttermilk and oil and pour over mixture of dry ingredients. Mix lightly.

Prepare a surface lightly covered with flour. Knead and roll dough on the flour-covered surface and then roll out dough to 3/4 inch thickness. Cut in 2 to 3 inch squares.

Bake at 450 degrees Fahrenheit for 10 to 12 minutes until golden brown.

QUICK AND EASY ROLLS

12 servings (1 mcg of VITAMIN K per serving.)

2	cups	Self rising flour
1/4	cup	Nonfat buttermilk
1/4	cup	Plus 2 tablespoons mayonnaise, home made Oil, olive or Canola, treated (See DIETARY TIP # 10.)

Combine first 3 ingredients, stirring until moistened.

Spoon batter into muffin pans coated with oil.

Bake at 375 degrees Fahrenheit for 12-15 minutes or until lightly browned.

EGG PANCAKES

2 servings (3 mcgs of VITAMIN K per serving.)

2	large	Eggs
1/2	cup	Milk
1/2	cup	Flour
1/2	teaspoon	Salt
1/2	stick	Butter (1/4 cup)

Mix eggs, milk, flour and salt until lumpy. Melt butter in pie plate. Pour batter into melted butter in pie plate. Bake in a 425 degree Fahrenheit oven for 20 minutes.

Serve with cooked apples, maple syrup, butter, powdered sugar, etc.

DATE OR RAISIN BRAN MUFFINS

12 servings (3.5 mcgs of VITAMIN K per serving.)

1	cup	Wheat or oat bran cereal
3/4	cup	Milk
1	cup	Unbleached all-purpose flour
2 1/2	teaspoon	Baking powder
1/2	teaspoon	Salt
1/4	cup	Granulated Sugar
1/2	cup	Seedless raisins *
1/2	cup	Chopped walnuts
1	Large	Egg
1/4	cup	Canola oil, treated (See DIETARY TIP # 10.)

*For Date Muffins, substitute finely chopped pitted dates.

Mix cereal and milk. Let stand a few minutes until most of the milk is absorbed.

Grease twelve 2 1/2-inch muffin cups. Heat oven to 400 degrees Fahrenheit.

Sift flour, baking powder, salt and sugar into a medium-sized bowl. Stir to mix well. Add dates or raisins and nuts. Toss to mix. Add egg and oil to soaked cereal and beat well with a fork. Pour into flour mixture and stir only until the dry ingredients are moistened. Batter will be lumpy. Drop batter into prepared pans, filling each cup half to two-thirds full.

Bake about 30 minutes, or until browned. Remove from pan and serve hot with butter and jelly or preserves.

CORN MEAL MUFFINS
12 servings (7 mcgs of VITAMIN K per muffin.)

1	cup	Unbleached all-purpose flour
4	teaspoons	Baking powder
2	tablespoons	Granulated sugar
1	teaspoons	Salt
1	cup	Yellow cornmeal
2	large	Eggs
1/4	cup	Canola oil, treated (See DIETARY TIP # 10.)

Grease 12, 2 1/2-inch muffin cups.

Heat oven to 425 degrees Fahrenheit.

Sift flour, baking powder, sugar and salt into medium-sized bowl. Add cornmeal and stir to mix well.

In small bowl, beat eggs with fork. Add milk and oil.

Add all at once to dry ingredients. Stir mixture only until dry ingredients are moistened. Batter will be lumpy.

Drop batter from a tablespoon into the prepared muffin cups, filling each cup 1/2 to 2/3 full.

Bake 15 to 20 minutes, or until golden brown. Remove and serve hot.

RICE PANCAKES
4 servings (Less than 2 mcgs of VITAMIN K per serving.)

1	cup	Cooked rice
2/3	cup	Milk
1/2	cup	Flour
1/4	teaspoon	Salt
1 or 2		Egg yolks
1or 2		Egg whites, beaten stiff
1	teaspoon	Baking powder

Mix all ingredients together, adding the beaten egg whites last. Bake on a greased griddle. You can add chopped and drained fresh fruit to batter if you like.

BACON AND ONION MUFFINS

12 servings (Less than 1 mcg of VITAMIN K per serving.)

1/2	pounds	Bacon, diced
1/4	cup	Chopped onion
2 1/4	cups	Unbleached flour, sifted
3	teaspoons	Baking powder
1/2	teaspoon	Baking soda
1/2	teaspoon	Salt
2	large	Eggs, slightly beaten
1/3	cup	Milk
1	cup	Dairy sour cream

Fry bacon in skillet until crisp. Remove with slotted spoon and drain on paper towels.

Sauté onion in 1 tablespoon bacon drippings until tender (do not brown). Set aside to cool.

Sift together flour, baking powder, baking soda and salt in large mixing bowl.

Combine eggs, milk and sour cream in a small bowl. Blend well.

Add all at once to dry ingredients, stirring just enough to moisten. Stir in bacon and sautéed onion. Spoon batter into greased 2 1/2-inch muffin-pan cups, fill 2/3 full.

Bake in 375 degree Fahrenheit oven 18 to 20 minutes or until golden brown. Serve hot with homemade jelly or jam.

SAUSAGE, EGGPLANT, BASIL AND TOMATO PIZZA

8 servings (13 mcg of VITAMIN K per serving.)

1/2	pound	Italian sausage, crumbled
1	medium	Eggplant, in 1/2 inch slices (about 1 1/4 cup)
1/3	cup	Onion, chopped
1	12 inch	Pizza crust
1/3	cup	Marinara sauce
1/4	cup	Parmesan, grated
1/2	cup	Mozzarella, shredded
1	medium	Tomato, diced (about 3/4 cup)
2	tablespoons	Basil, fresh, thinly sliced

Cook sausage for 6 to 8 minutes and set aside.

Add onion to skillet and cook until onion begins to brown, 5 to 8 minutes, cover and cook 5 minutes until tender. Meanwhile, (peel the eggplant if you wish) brush the eggplant with treated olive oil on both sides. Broil in broiler until brown on both sides, turning once.

Spread baked crust with sauce. Top with the sausage and onion mixture, eggplant, cheeses, tomatoes and basil.

Bake 10 minutes at 400 degrees Fahrenheit.

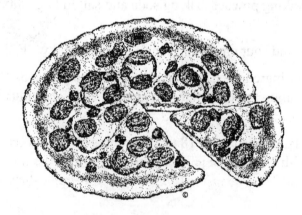

JUMBO POPOVERS

6 servings (Less than 1 mcg of VITAMIN K per serving.)

2	large	Eggs
1	cup	Non-fat milk
1	cup	Sifted flour
1/2	teaspoon	Salt

Butter 6 six-ounce custard cups with straight sides (popovers rise better in straight-sided container).

Beat eggs slightly with rotary beater. Add other ingredients. Continue beating briskly 1 to 2 minutes. Mixture will be smooth and thin.

Pour into custard cups, about 1/2 full. Place cups on cookie sheet, not touching. Cook at 400 for 50 minutes or until puffed up and golden brown (do NOT peek until they are done - this may cause them to fall).

SMOKED SALMON-AND-CHIVE SANDWICHES

6 servings (15 mcgs of VITAMIN K per serving.)

12	slices	Thinly sliced pumpernickel bread
6	ounces	Thinly sliced smoked salmon
8	ounces	Cream cheese, soft
4	ounces	Butter, soft
1	tablespoon	Grated lemon zest
		Salt and pepper
3	tablespoons	Fresh chives, finely chopped

Beat together cream cheese and butter until smooth and light. Beat in lemon zest and salt and pepper to taste. Stir in chives.

Lay out 6 slices of the bread. Carefully spread with half the filling. Place the salmon, overlapping if necessary, in an even layer over the filling. Spread with the remaining filling and top with the remaining slices of bread.

Trim off the crusts and cut the sandwiches into quarters.

ORANGE SPREAD

4 servings (2 mcgs of VITAMIN K per serving.)

3/4	cup	Orange
8	ounces	Cream cheese
1	tablespoon	Honey
1	tablespoon	Pecans
4		Bagels

Grate orange rind. Peel, seed and chop orange. Soften cream cheese.
Chop pecans. Combine and serve on bagels.

TUNA BUNS

8 servings (6 mcgs of VITAMIN K per serving.)

2		Hard cooked eggs, chopped
6 1/2	ounces	(1 can) Tuna, drained, water pack
4	ounces	Shredded cheddar cheese
1/4	cup	Chopped green pepper
2	tablespoons	Finely chopped onion
1/2	teaspoon	Prepared mustard
1/2	cup	Mayonnaise, homemade (See Recipe Index.)
8		Hamburger buns, split

Mix eggs, tuna, cheese, green pepper, onion, mustard and mayonnaise.
Fill buns with tuna mixture. Wrap each bun individually in aluminum foil.
Place on cookie sheet and heat them in the oven at 350 degrees Fahrenheit
for about 20 minutes.

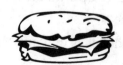
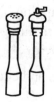

EARLY BIRD BUTTERMILK PANCAKES
4 servings (5 mcgs of VITAMIN K per serving.)

1 1/2	cups	Flour
1	tablespoon	Sugar
1/2	teaspoon	Salt
2 1/4	teaspoons	Baking powder
1/2	cup	Buttermilk
2/3	cup	Milk
1	large	Egg (beaten)
2	tablespoons	Canola oil, treated (See DIETARY TIP # 10.)
		Canola oil, treated, for pan
1/2	cup	Milk for thinning as needed

Sift together the flour, sugar, salt, and baking powder. Beat together the buttermilk, milk, beaten egg and oil. Pour the liquid into the dry ingredients and stir until well mixed. A few small lumps in the mixture will cook out.

The first pancake is a test pancake. The batter should be thin for pancakes. So thin the batter, if necessary, with milk (not buttermilk). The pan should be lightly oiled and hot enough to make a sprinkling of water dance, not just sit and sizzle.

Ladle about 1/8 cup of the batter into the hot pan. When the top of the pancake is full of bubbles and the bottom is golden, turn the pancake. Cook on the second side until done. Makes 15 (4 inch) pancakes.

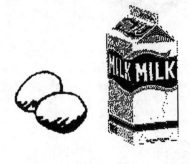

BLUEBERRY BUTTERMILK PANCAKES
4 servings (5 mcgs of VITAMIN K per serving.)

1	cup	Flour
1/2	teaspoon	Salt
1	teaspoons	Baking soda
1	cup	Buttermilk
2	large	Eggs, slightly beaten
1	cup	Blueberries, washed and dried

Blend flour, salt and baking soda.

In separate bowl, combine buttermilk, eggs and butter.

Stir the two mixtures together just long enough to blend them, but do not overbeat.

Fold in blueberries. Heat 2-3 tablespoons of butter on a griddle or large skillet over medium heat.

Spoon out 3-4 tablespoons of batter for each pancake. Cook until the bubbles that form on top begin to pop, then flip. Cook a minute or so more, then remove pancakes to heated dish.

Serve with butter and syrup.

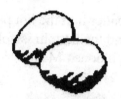

APPLE PANCAKE PUFF

4 servings (2 mcgs of VITAMIN K per serving.)

1	tablespoon	Plus 1 teaspoon butter
3	small	Apples, peeled, cored & cut into 1/4 inch thick slices
2	tablespoons	Dark raisins
3	tablespoons	Granulated sugar
2	tablespoons	Orange juice
1	teaspoons	Cinnamon
2	large	Eggs
1/2	cup	Skim milk
1/4	cup	Plus 2 tablespoons flour
1	teaspoons	Vanilla extract

In a heavy, medium sized, oven proof skillet, melt 2 teaspoons of the butter. Add apples, raisins, 1 tablespoon sugar, orange juice and cinnamon. Cook, stirring frequently, 6 to 8 minutes, until apples are just tender. Remove apples and raisins to bowl.

Preheat oven to 425 degrees Fahrenheit.

In a small bowl (with an electric mixer) beat eggs until foamy. Gradually add milk, flour, sugar and the vanilla, beat 2 minutes longer, until batter is smooth.

Add remaining 2 teaspoons of butter to the same skillet. Place in oven to melt, about 1 minute. Pour batter into skillet and bake 10 minutes.

Remove from oven and spoon apple mixture into center of pancake. Return to oven and bake 12-15 minutes longer until puffed and golden. Cut into quarters.

GARLIC BREAD
6 servings (6 mcgs of VITAMIN K per serving.)

1	loaf	Sourdough or Italian bread
		Butter
3/4	cup	Mayonnaise, homemade (See Recipe Index.)
3/4	cup	Parmesan cheese, fresh grated
1	tablespoon	Garlic, minced

Cut bread horizontally in half. Butter and brown each half under the broiler.

Mix remaining ingredients and spread each half evenly with 1/2 of topping mixture.

Bake at 425 degrees Fahrenheit for about 15 to 20 minutes or until crust is well browned.

Cut in wedges and serve hot or at room temperature.

POTATO CRACKERS
20 servings (8 mcgs of VITAMIN K for the whole recipe.)

3/4	cup	Rolled oats
3/4	cup	Flour
1/3	cup	Butter
2	cups	Potatoes, cooked and mashed

Combine oats and flour in a bowl. Rub in butter with fingertips, then knead in mashed potatoes to form a stiff dough.

Carefully roll out on a floured board and cut out thin rounds using a cookie cutter or upside-down glass.

Cook on greased trays at 350 degrees Fahrenheit for 20 minutes or until crackers are crisp and lightly browned.

BASIC PANCAKES

4 servings (1.5 mcgs of VITAMIN K per serving.)

3/4	cup	Flour
1/2	teaspoon	Salt
1 1/2	teaspoon	Sugar
1	teaspoons	Baking powder
1	large	Egg
1 1/2	teaspoon	Canola oil, treated (See DIETARY TIP # 10.)
5/8	cups	Milk (you can use low-fat)

Sift the dry ingredients together into a bowl.

Combine the egg, oil and milk together in another bowl, then stir the wet ingredients into the dry ingredients until batter is just smooth.

Lightly grease a large skillet or griddle. When hot, ladle the batter onto the griddle. (Usually, 3 pancakes fit in a large skillet.)

Adjust heat to medium-high. When bubbles appear on the surface of the pancake, usually after 2 to 3 minutes, lift with a spatula to see that the underside is browned. Turn and cook the second side until browned, about 1 1/2 to 2 minutes. Serve hot with butter and syrup.

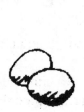
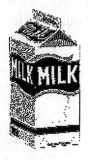

SCOTTISH SCONES

8 servings (1 mcg of VITAMIN K per serving.)

2	cups	Flour
1	teaspoons	Salt
1	teaspoon	Baking soda
2	teaspoons	Cream of tartar
3	tablespoons	Butter, room temperature
1	large	Egg, room temperature, lightly beaten
1/2	cup	Buttermilk, room temperature

In bowl, mix flour, salt, baking soda and cream of tartar. Stir thoroughly.

With fingers, rub the butter into the dry ingredients. Gradually stir beaten egg and buttermilk into the flour mix. If it is a bit too moist and sticks to hands, add a bit of flour.

Turn the dough onto a lightly floured work surface and knead as little as possible to achieve a soft, pliable dough ball.

Divide dough into 2 equal parts. Flatten each with the knuckles into a round disc (about 6 inches in diameter and 1/2 inch thick). Prick about a dozen times with fork. Then cut in four sections each.

Bake on lightly greased baking sheet until tan. Bake at 375 degrees Fahrenheit for about 15 minutes. You can add 1/2 cup raisins or currants if you wish.

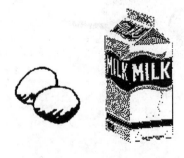

IRISH SODA BREAD

8 servings (1 mcg of VITAMIN K per serving.)

3	tablespoons	Butter, soft
2 1/2	cups	Flour
2	tablespoons	Sugar
1	teaspoon	Baking soda
1	teaspoon	Baking powder
1/2	teaspoon	Salt
1/3	cup	Raisins (optional)
3/4	cup	Buttermilk

Heat oven to 375 degrees Fahrenheit. Cut butter into flour, sugar, baking soda, baking powder & salt until mixture resembles fine crumbs. Stir in raisins and enough buttermilk to make a soft dough.

Turn onto lightly floured surface. Knead until smooth, about 1 to 2 minutes. Shape into round loaf, about 6 1/2 inches in diameter. Place on greased baking sheet.

Cut an X about 1/4-inch through the center of the loaf with a floured knife. Bake until golden brown, 35 to 45 minutes.

Brush with butter if desired. Delicious warm, or cool to slice more easily.

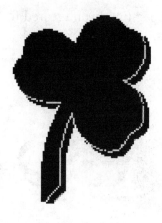

APPLESAUCE BANANA BREAD

12 servings (Less than 1 mcg of VITAMIN K per serving.)

2 1/2	cups	All-purpose flour
2	teaspoons	Baking powder
1	teaspoon	Baking soda
1	teaspoon	Ground cinnamon
1/2	cup	Applesauce
1	cup	Granulated sugar
3		Egg whites
4	large	Bananas, very ripe, peeled and mashed (2 cups)
1	teaspoon	Vanilla extract
		Butter or treated Canola oil for greasing pan

Preheat oven to 350 degrees Fahrenheit.

Coat an 8 by 4 by 3 inch loaf pan with butter.

Combine flour, baking powder, baking soda, and cinnamon. Set aside.

In a large mixing bowl, whisk together apple sauce, sugar, egg whites, banana and vanilla. Add flour mixture all at once and stir gently to blend.

Pour batter into prepared loaf pan and bake for 50-60 minutes or until knife inserted into the center comes out clean. Cool bread completely before slicing.

NOTE: Loaf can be wrapped tightly and stored for up to one week or frozen for up to 2 months.

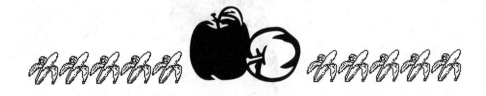

BEEF

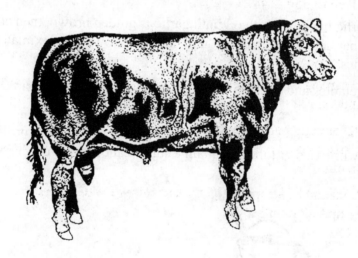

BEEF STIR FRY

4 Servings (VITAMIN K content of beef stir fry (without rice or tortilla) = 4 mcg per cup)

3	cups	Lean steak, cut into small pieces, either thin strips or small cubes, with fat trimmed
1	clove	Minced garlic
2	cups	Sliced onions
1 1/2	cups	Sliced tomatoes
2	teaspoons	Canola or olive oil, treated (See DIETARY TIP # 10.)
1	teaspoon	Vinegar
1/8	teaspoon	Salt
1/4	teaspoon	Black pepper

Sauté garlic in skillet with oil until garlic is golden brown, then add steak, salt, pepper, and vinegar. Cook until steak is brown, approximately 5 to 10 minutes.

Add vegetables and cook until onions and tomatoes are at desired tenderness.

This recipe is especially good served with white rice or on a tortilla. Neither white rice or tortilla contain a significant amount of VITAMIN K.

BEEF STROGANOFF

8 servings (1 mcg of VITAMIN K per serving.)

1 1/2	pounds	Beef fillet, or sirloin
		Salt and pepper, to taste
3	tablespoons	Butter
1	can	Cream of mushroom soup, low fat **OR**
1 1/2	cups	Mushroom Cream Sauce (See Recipe Index.)
1	cup	Beef stock, hot
1	teaspoon	Mustard, Dijon preferred
2	tablespoons	Catsup
1/2	cup	Onion, sliced or chopped
2	teaspoons	Worcestershire sauce
1/2	cup	Sour cream or plain yogurt
3	tablespoons	Brandy
1	tablespoon	Hungarian paprika

Remove all the fat and gristle from the meat. Cut into narrow strips about 2 inches long and 1/2 inch thick. Season the strips with salt, pepper and paprika.

In a saucepan, melt 1 1/2 tablespoon of butter. Add the meat strips and brown. Remove the beef from the pan and keep warm. Add the other 1 1/2 tablespoon of butter, add the onion and sauté until golden.

Put the beef back into the pan. Add the brandy and cook for two minutes on medium heat. Add the hot beef stock and the cream of mushroom soup. Stir until well blended. Stir in mustard and Worcestershire sauce.

Add the sour cream and heat over a brisk flame for 3 minutes. Serve sauce and meat over buttered noodles.

MEATLOAF

4 servings (VITAMIN K for entire loaf = 154 mcgs or almost 40 mcgs per serving.)

1	pound	Lean ground beef
1/4	cup	Homemade bread crumbs
1/2	cup	Tomato paste
1/4	cup	Chopped onions
1/4	cup	Green peppers
1	cup	Fresh, chopped tomatoes
1/2	teaspoon	Mustard
1/2	teaspoon	Black pepper
2	cloves	Minced garlic
1/4	cup	Chopped scallions

Mix all ingredients together and bake at 325 degrees Fahrenheit for 1 hour.

BREADED VEAL CUTLET (WEINERSCHNITZEL)

6 servings (Less than 1 mcg of VITAMIN K per serving.)

2	pounds	Veal steak, 1/2 inch thick
		Salt and pepper
		Crackers, crushed or: bread crumbs
1	large	Egg, beaten
		Lemon juice
6		Eggs, fried

Cut the veal steak in pieces for serving. Sprinkle with salt and pepper, dip in cracker or bread crumbs, then in beaten egg, then again in crumbs. Let stand a few minutes then fry on both sides.

Sprinkle with lemon juice and garnish with a fried egg per portion.

BEEF TACOS

6 servings (34 mcgs of VITAMIN K per serving or 17 mcgs per taco.)

1	pound	Ground beef
3/4	cup	Chopped onion, medium
1/2	cup	Green pepper, chopped
1 1/2	cups	Potato cooked and diced
1	cup	Tomatoes chopped
1/2	teaspoon	Sugar
1	tablespoon	Chili powder
1	teaspoon	Coriander
		Salt and pepper to taste
1/2	cup	Olives, black chopped
12		Pre-shaped taco shells
1	cup	Tomato, chopped
1/8	cup	ITALIAN HERB DRESSING (See Recipe Index)
4	ounces	Cheddar cheese, grated

Sauté the beef, green pepper and onion until meat is brown and veggies are translucent. Add the potato, tomatoes, sugar, chili powder, coriander, salt and pepper and stir to blend, cooking a few minutes more.

Mix in the olives. Cook for about 10 minutes more, stirring constantly.

Put pre-shaped taco shells in oven and heat, to crisp them.

Place a heaping tablespoon of meat mixture in each shell and stuff with tomato and cheese that have been tossed with ITALIAN HERB DRESSING. Top with sour cream.

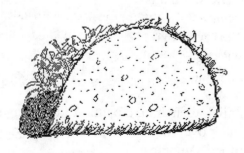

CROCK POT CHILI CON CARNE

6 servings (12 mcgs of VITAMIN K per serving.)

1	pound	Lean ground beef
1	small	Onion, chopped
1	teaspoon	Salt
1		Bay leaf
1	teaspoon	Chili powder
1	teaspoon	Worcestershire sauce
16	ounces	Tomato sauce
2	cans (16oz)	Kidney beans, drained

In skillet (or crock pot with browning unit) break up beef with fork and cook until lightly browned. Pour off excess fat.

In crock pot, combine meat with onion, salt, chili powder, bay leaf, Worcestershire sauce, tomato sauce, and kidney beans. Cover and cook on high for 2 to 3 hours. Remove bay leaf.

HAMBURG CASSEROLE

5 Servings (VITAMIN K content = 18 mcg per cup)

1	cup	Lean ground beef
1	cup	Diced green pepper
1/2	teaspoon	Black pepper
1	cup	Diced carrots
1	cup	Diced onions
1	cup	Diced celery
3 1/2	cups	Diced tomatoes
1/4	teaspoon	Salt
1	cup	Frozen peas
1	cup	Rice
1 1/2	cups	Water

Brown the beef in a skillet, then drain the fat. Add the remainder of the ingredients, mix and cook over medium heat until boiling. Cover skillet and cook on low heat for 35 minutes.

TEXAS CHILI

8 servings (12 mcgs of VITAMIN K per serving. Add a 16 ounce can of Navy beans and increase the VITAMIN K count to 13 mcgs per serving)

2	tablespoons	Canola or olive oil, treated (See DIETARY TIP # 10.)
2	pounds	Ground beef
2	medium	Onions, chopped
2	cloves	Garlic, finely chopped
28	ounces	Tomatoes, whole, peeled
12	ounces	Beer
5	tablespoons	Chili powder
2		Jalapeno chili, seeded and chopped
1	tablespoon	Cumin
2	teaspoons	Paprika
1	teaspoon	Sugar
		Cheddar cheese, shredded
		Onion, chopped
		Sour cream (low fat is fine)

Heat oil in 6-quart saucepan. Add ground beef, onions and garlic and sauté until meat is browned. Stir in next 7 ingredients and bring to boil over medium-high heat. Reduce heat to medium-low and simmer, uncovered, about 45-55 minutes. Taste and season with salt, pepper and cayenne pepper, if desired.

Ladle into bowls. Garnish with cheese, chopped raw onion and sour cream if desired.

You can add canned navy beans to the pot during the last 20 minutes of cooking time if desired.

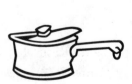

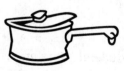

ENCHILADA PIE

8 servings (1 mcg of VITAMIN K per serving.)

1	pound	Lean ground chuck
1/2	cup	Chopped onion
4	ounces	Tomato sauce
1	teaspoon	Chili powder
1/2	teaspoon	Cumin
1/4	teaspoon	Salt
1/4	teaspoon	Pepper
4		Corn tortillas
3/4	cup	Shredded cheese (American, cheddar or Monterey Jack.)
1/2	cup	Water
		Oil, olive or Canola, treated (See DIETARY TIP # 10.)

Cook beef and onion until browned.

Stir in tomato sauce and seasonings and cook until heated.

Layer tortillas, meat sauce and cheese in a 2 quart casserole coated with oil. Pour water over top. Cover and bake in the oven at 400 degrees Fahrenheit for 20 minutes. (If you fry the tortillas in oil before adding to this dish they will stay together more. It does add the extra fat.)

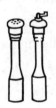

VEAL PARMIGIANA

6 servings (3 mcgs of VITAMIN K per serving.)

1	large	Egg, beaten
1/2	teaspoon	Salt
1/4	teaspoon	Pepper
1/4	cup	Soft bread crumbs
1	tablespoon	Grated parmesan cheese
1	pound	Thin veal cutlets cut into 6 serving size pieces
8	ounces	Tomato sauce
2	ounces	Mozzarella cheese
2	tablespoons	Canola or olive oil, treated (See DIETARY TIP # 10.)

Combine egg, salt and pepper and beat with a wire whisk until blended.

Combine bread crumbs and Parmesan cheese, stirring well.

Dip veal into egg mixture, and dredge in bread crumbs mixture.

Put the oil into a large skillet. Sauté veal until golden brown. Transfer veal to shallow baking dish. Pour tomato sauce over veal, and top with cheese slices.

Bake at 350 degrees Fahrenheit for 15-20 minutes. Serve immediately.

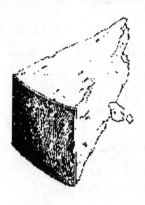

VEAL MARSALA

6 servings (20 mcgs of VITAMIN K per serving.)

1	pound	Thin veal, cut in medallion sized pieces
1 1/4	cups	Self-rising flour
10	tablespoons	Butter
1/4	cup	Green onions, sliced
1/4	cup	Stock
3	cups	Mushrooms, sliced
1/4	cup	Dry Marsala wine
		Salt and pepper
		Lemon slices

Pound veal thin and dredge in flour. Shake off excess. In pan, melt the butter over medium to high heat and sauté veal until golden brown. Remove to a platter and keep warm.

In the same pan, add the stock to deglaze the pan. Add onions, mushrooms, and wine. Simmer to reduce sauce to half.

Pour sauce over veal and garnish with lemons.

VEAL NORMANDE

4 servings (1 mcg of VITAMIN K per serving.)

1 1/2	tablespoons	Butter
1 1/2	tablespoons	Oil, olive or Canola, treated (See DIETARY TIP # 10.)
6		Veal cutlets, thinly sliced or 6 pieces of boneless chicken (preferably breasts)
1/2	cup	Shallots, chopped
5	tablespoons	Brandy
2/3	cup	Milk
1		Tart apple peeled sliced
		Wild rice, freshly cooked

Melt butter with oil in a large skillet over medium-high heat. Add veal and brown, turning once. Transfer to platter.

Add brandy and shallots to skillet and stir, scraping up any browned bits clinging to bottom of pan. Blend in soup and milk.

Return veal to pan with peeled apple. Reduce heat and simmer, stirring once or twice, until heated through. Serve over rice.

SAUCY MEATLOAF

8 servings (3 mcgs of VITAMIN K per serving.)

1	cup	Ketchup
2	tablespoons	Dijon mustard
1 1/2	tablespoons	Brown sugar
2	pounds	Ground chuck, course grind
1/2	cup	Onions, dice
1/2	teaspoon	Garlic, mince
1/4	cup	Green pepper, dice
3/4	cup	Bread crumbs
2	large	Eggs (or 1/2 cup egg substitute)
1 1/2	teaspoon	Salt
1/2	teaspoon	Pepper

Combine ketchup, mustard and sugar for a sauce.

Mix meat and remaining ingredients. Pat in loaf shape and turn out into a baking pan with sides. Put 2/3 cup of sauce on top of loaf. Bake in a preheated 350 degree Fahrenheit oven about 45 minutes to an hour or until a quick-read thermometer says 130.

Serve with remaining sauce.

VEAL OSCAR WITH SHRIMP

1 serving (20 mcgs of VITAMIN K per serving with asparagus. Less than 1 mcg of VITAMIN K per serving without asparagus.)

3	ounces	Veal
		Salt, pepper
		Flour
		Oil, Canola or olive, treated (See DIETARY TIP # 10.)
		SAUCE BERNAISE OR HOLLANDAISE, (See Recipe Index.)
2		Green asparagus spears
1/2	cup	Shrimp, peeled, deveined and chopped
1/4	cup	Sliced mushrooms
1/4	cup	Chopped onions

Season veal with salt and pepper, dust with flour and sauté 2-3 minutes on both sides. Place veal on plate and cover with sauce Bernaise or Hollandaise. Place 2 asparagus spears on top of veal one inch apart and fill space with shrimp mixture.

SHRIMP MIXTURE: Sauté onions and mushrooms in butter until tender, add shrimp, sauté 5 more minutes, season to taste. Can also use crab.

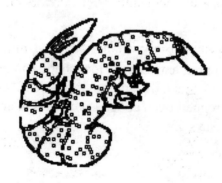

VEAL CHILI

2 servings (30 mcgs of VITAMIN K per serving.)

1	tablespoon	Canola or olive oil, treated (See DIETARY TIP # 10.)
1/2	cup	Diced onion
1/2		Jalapeno pepper, minced
1/2	pound	Ground veal
1 1/2	cups	Canned tomatoes with liquid, chopped
1/2	cup	Tomato sauce
1	tablespoon	Chili powder
1	teaspoon	Dry mustard
		Salt and pepper
1/4	teaspoon	Basil, fresh minced
1/4	teaspoon	Oregano, fresh minced
4	ounces	Drained canned red kidney beans
2	tablespoons	Dry white wine
1	teaspoon	Lemon juice

Sauté onion and jalapeno pepper over medium heat for about 2 minutes.

Add veal and cook for 5-7 minutes until pink color is gone.

Add tomatoes, reserved liquid, tomato sauce and seasonings. Stir to combine. Reduce heat to low and let simmer until flavors blend, about 5 minutes.

Add remaining ingredients and stir to combine. Cook 15 minutes longer. Serve.

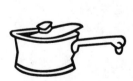
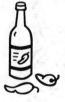
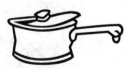

VEAL PICCATA
4 servings (Less than 1 mcg of VITAMIN K per serving.)

1/4	cup	Flour
1	pound	Leg of veal, sliced very thin and cut into 3x4 inch pieces
1/4	cup	Canola or olive oil, treated (See DIETARY TIP # 10.)
2	tablespoons	Butter
		Juice of 1 lemon
1/4	cup	Dry white wine
1		Lemon
		Salt and pepper

Lightly flour veal on both sides. Shake off excess. In a large heavy skillet, heat the oil and butter. When bubbling, add veal and sauté about 2 minutes on each side. When the veal is nearly cooked, sprinkle with lemon juice. Remove veal from the pan and keep warm.

Add wine to the pan and deglaze over high heat, stirring constantly. Reduce liquid to about 3 tablespoons.

Pour sauce over veal. Slice the lemon to paper thinness and put a slice on each veal scallop. Sprinkle with salt and pepper.

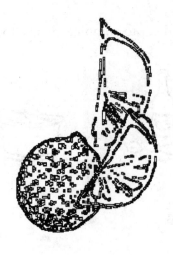

VEAL SCALOPPINI

6 servings (1 mcg of VITAMIN K per serving.)

1 1/2	pounds	Veal steak, 1/2 inch thick
1/4	cup	Flour
1/4	cup	Canola oil, treated (See DIETARY TIP # 10.)
1/2	cup	Onion, sliced thin
1		Bell pepper, cut in strips
12	ounces	Chicken broth
1/4	pound	Mushrooms
1	tablespoon	Butter

MARINADE/SAUCE

1	teaspoon	Salt
1	teaspoon	Paprika
1/2	cup	Canola or olive oil, treated (See DIETARY TIP # 10.)
1/4	cup	Lemon juice
1	clove	Garlic, split
1	teaspoon	Prepared mustard
1/4	teaspoon	Nutmeg
1/2	teaspoon	Sugar

In sauce pan, combine all sauce ingredients and bring to a boil.

Pound veal with meat hammer to 1/4 inch thick and lay flat in baking dish. Pour sauce over veal and turn to coat thoroughly. Let stand 15 minutes. Remove garlic.

Remove veal from sauce and dredge in flour. Brown in hot oil in heavy skillet. Add onion and green pepper. Combine chicken broth with sauce and pour over veal. Cover and cook slowly in oven preheated to 350 degrees Fahrenheit until veal is very tender, about 40 minutes.

Clean and slice mushrooms. Brown lightly in butter. Place mushrooms on the veal and ladle sauce over top. Cook 5 minutes more. May be served over noodles.

OVEN-BAKED BOURGUIGNONNE

8 servings (5 mcg of VITAMIN K per serving.)

2	pounds	Boneless beef chuck cut into 1 inch cubes as with stew meat.
1/4	cup	Unbleached all-purpose flour
1 1/3	cups	Sliced carrots
14 1/2	ounces	Tomatoes, should be whole peeled tomatoes, undrained and chopped or use crushed tomatoes
1		Bay leaf
1	envelope	Soup mix (Onion or Beefy Onion soup mix.)
1/2	cup	Red wine
8	ounces	Mushrooms
2	cups	Cooked rice OR
8	ounces	Medium or broad egg noodles

In a 2-quart casserole, toss beef with flour. Add carrots, tomatoes, bay leaf, and mushrooms then add beefy onion recipe soup mix blended with wine.

Cook at 250 degrees Fahrenheit for 7 hours or until beef is tender. Remove bay leaf.

Meanwhile, cook noodles or rice according to package directions.

To serve, arrange Bourguignonne over noodles.

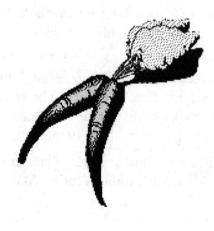

STEAK PARMIGIANA
6 servings (8 mcgs of VITAMIN K per serving.)

1 1/2	pounds	Top round steak,1/2 inch thick
1/3	cup	Bread crumbs, dry
1/3	cup	Parmesan cheese, grated
1		Egg, beaten
1/3	cup	Canola oil, treated (See DIETARY TIP # 10.)
1	cup	Onion, chopped
8	ounces	Tomato sauce
16	ounces	Tomatoes, stewed
		Salt and pepper to taste
1	teaspoon	Basil, fresh minced
1/2	teaspoon	Oregano, fresh minced
1 1/2	cups	Mozzarella cheese, grated

Trim excess fat from steak and cut into 6 pieces. Pound each piece with a heavy mallet to 1/4-inch thickness.

Combine bread crumbs and Parmesan cheese. Dip each piece of meat in beaten egg and then in the crumb mixture.

Heat oil in a large skillet, brown steak well on both sides. Remove steak to paper towels to drain.

Add onion, tomato sauce, stewed tomatoes, salt, pepper, basil and oregano to skillet, stir to combine. Bring mixture to a boil, lower heat and simmer, uncovered, 30 minutes.

Spoon 5 tablespoons cooked tomato mixture into the bottom of a 13x9x2-inch baking dish (enough to lightly cover bottom of dish). Place steak on top of sauce in a single layer, pour remaining sauce over steak.

Bake in preheated 350 degrees Fahrenheit oven for 1 hour.

Remove from oven and sprinkle with cheese.

Bake 15 minutes longer, or until cheese is melted. Serve with spaghetti or polenta.

VEAL SALTIMBOCCA A LA ROMANA

6 servings (Less than 1 mcg of VITAMIN K per serving.)

3 1/2	pounds	Veal steak, cut 1/2 inch thick
1/2	teaspoon	Chopped fresh sage
1/2	teaspoon	Freshly ground black pepper
1/4	pound	Prosciutto ham, sliced paper-thin
4	tablespoons	Butter
2	tablespoons	Olive or Canola oil, treated (See DIETARY TIP # 10.)
3	tablespoons	Flour
3/4	cup	Dry Marsala wine

Preheat oven to 325 degrees Fahrenheit.

Bone and trim the fat from the meat. Pound with a meat mallet to 1/8 inch thickness. Rub on one side with the sage and pepper. Cut into 4 to 5 inch squares.

Distribute the ham over the seasoned side of the veal pieces. Carefully roll up each piece and secure with wooden toothpicks.

Heat the butter and oil together in a large skillet over high heat. Brown the veal rolls on all sides.

Remove to a 13 1/2 inch by 9 inch by 2 inch baking dish, reserving the pan drippings.

Stir the flour into the drippings. Stir in 1-1/2 cups water and the Marsala and bring to a boil. Pour over the veal rolls.

Cover the baking dish with aluminum foil and bake in preheated oven for 35 minutes or until tender.

Serve. Smoked or boiled ham may be used if prosciutto is unavailable.

ITALIAN MEAT LOAF

4 servings (5 mcg of VITAMIN K per serving.)

1 1/4	pounds	Beef, ground
1		Egg, beaten
1/4	cup	Tomato sauce or tomato puree
6	tablespoons	Soft bread crumbs
1/2	teaspoon	Fresh oregano leaves
1	clove	Garlic, crushed
		Salt and pepper to taste
2 1/2	ounces	Salami, chopped
3	ounces	Mozzarella cheese, chopped

In a bowl, combine egg, tomato sauce, bread crumbs, oregano, garlic, salt and pepper. Add ground beef. Mix well.

Place meat on foil. Shape into a 7x9 inch rectangle. Evenly sprinkle salami over top. Sprinkle cheese over salami, leaving a narrow margin around edges.

Beginning from the 7 inch end, roll the meat jelly roll fashion, using foil to help you roll. Press to seal edges. Place loaf seam side down in a greased baking pan.

Bake at 350 degree Fahrenheit for 1 hour or until done. Drain fat. Slice. Serve immediately.

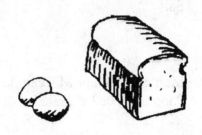

UPSIDE DOWN PIZZA
8 servings (5 mcgs of VITAMIN K per serving.)

FILLING

1 1/2	pounds	Lean ground beef
1	cup	Onion, chopped
1	cup	Green pepper, chopped
1	clove	Garlic
1/2	teaspoon	Oregano, fresh minced
1	dash	Salt
1/2	cup	Water
1/8	teaspoon	Hot pepper sauce
1	Package	Spaghetti sauce mix (1.5oz)

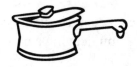

BATTER

1	cup	Milk
1	cup	Flour
1	tablespoon	Olive or Canola oil, treated (See DIETARY TIP # 10.)
2		Eggs
1/2	teaspoon	Salt

MISCELLANEOUS

7	ounces	Monterey Jack or Mozzarella cheese slices
1/2	cup	Parmesan cheese, grated

Pre-heat oven to 400 degrees Fahrenheit.

FILLING

In a large skillet, brown the beef and drain. Stir in onion, green pepper, garlic, oregano, salt, water, hot pepper sauce, tomato sauce and sauce mix. Simmer about 10 minutes stirring occasionally.

BATTER

In a bowl, combine milk, oil and eggs, beat 1 minute on medium speed. Add flour and salt, beat 2 minutes or until smooth.

ASSEMBLY

Pour hot meat mixture into 13x9 pan, top with cheese slices. Pour batter over cheese, covering filling completely. Sprinkle with parmesan cheese. Bake at 400 degrees Fahrenheit for 25-30 minutes or until puffed and brown.

To serve, cut in squares and lift out with a spatula.

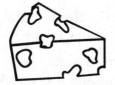 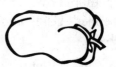

GARLIC MEATBALLS
4 servings (6 mcgs of VITAMIN K per serving.)

1 1/2	cups	Onions
2	tablespoons	Butter
1	pound	Lean ground beef
3	cloves	Garlic, minced
1	cup	Bread crumbs
1	teaspoon	Salt
1/4	teaspoon	Pepper
1	tablespoon	Olive oil, treated (See DIETARY TIP # 10.)
2	cups	Tomato juice
2	teaspoons	Lemon juice
2	teaspoons	Sugar
1	tablespoon	Cornstarch
2	tablespoons	Cold water

Mince 1/2 cup onion and reserve. Slice remaining onion. In a large skillet, melt the butter. Add sliced onion and cook over medium heat, stirring often, until golden brown, about 8 minutes. Transfer to a plate and set the skillet aside.

In a medium bowl, combine beef, minced onion, garlic, bread crumbs, salt and pepper. Using about 2 tablespoons for each, form into 12 large meatballs.

In the same skillet the onions were cooked in, heat the oil. Add meatballs and cook over medium high heat, turning often, until browned all over, about 8 minutes.

Return cooked onions to skillet. Stir in tomato juice, lemon juice, and sugar. Bring to a boil, reduce heat to low, cover and simmer until meatballs are cooked through, about 10 minutes. In a small bowl dissolve cornstarch in 2 tablespoons cold water. Stir into tomato sauce and cook, stirring, until thickened, about 1 minute. (If your tomato juice is very thick, you may not need to do this last step.)

POULTRY

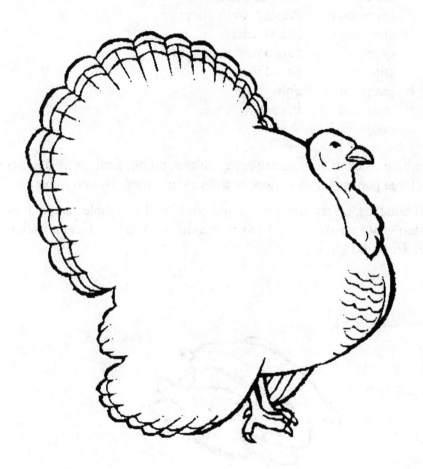

CHICKEN RAGOUT
6 servings (VITAMIN K content = 5 mcg per cup)

5	cups	Chicken pieces with skin and fat removed
1	clove	Minced garlic
1/2	cup	Diced onion
2	cups	Chopped tomatoes
1	teaspoon	Parsley, fresh chopped
1/4	cup	Diced celery
2	cups	Diced peeled potatoes
1	cup	Diced carrots
1 1/2	teaspoon	Salt
1/2	teaspoon	Pepper
1	cup	Water

Combine chicken, tomatoes, parsley, water, onion, garlic, salt, and pepper in a large pan and cook on low heat for 30 minutes. Remove chicken.

Add potatoes, celery, and carrots and cook until vegetables are at desired tenderness (approximately 10 to 15 minutes). Add the chicken back to the pan. Heat and serve.

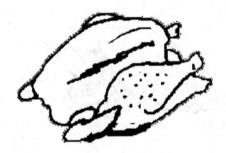

CHICKEN-FILLED TORTILLAS

5 servings (VITAMIN K content = 9 mcg per cup of chicken mixture with cheese. Tortillas contain negligible amounts of VITAMIN K)

1	tablespoon	Canola or olive oil, treated (See DIETARY TIP # 10.)
1/2	cup	Chopped onion
2	cups	Ground boneless, skinless chicken
1	cup	Grated mozzarella cheese or cheddar cheese
1/2	teaspoon	Salt
1/2	cup	Finely chopped tomato
1	clove	Finely minced garlic
1	cup	Chopped green pepper

Sauté chicken in Canola oil on low heat until chicken is white. Add vegetables and garlic to skillet and cook until vegetables are tender. Allow to cool, then mix in cheese.

Serve on flour tortillas (can be corn or white flour tortillas)

CROCKPOT BAKED CHICKEN BREASTS

4 servings (4 mcgs of VITAMIN K per serving.)

2		Whole chicken breasts
2	teaspoons	Butter
1	can	Cream chicken soup
1/2	cup	Dry sherry
1	teaspoon	Fresh rosemary, minced
1	teaspoon	Worcestershire sauce
1/4	teaspoon	Garlic powder
4	ounces	Canned, drained mushrooms

Put chicken breasts in bottom of crock pot. In a bowl, mix other ingredients and then pour over chicken. Cover and cook on low 5-7 hours. Serve over rice or baked potatoes.

JAMAICAN JERK CHICKEN

8 servings (VITAMIN K content = 10 mcg per cup)

3	pounds	Boneless, skinless chicken pieces
3/4	teaspoon	Ground cinnamon
2	teaspoons	Black pepper
1	tablespoon	Chopped hot pepper
1	teaspoon	Fresh oregano
1	teaspoon	Fresh thyme
1/2	teaspoon	Salt
6	cloves	Minced garlic
1	cup	Finely chopped onion
1/4	cup	Vinegar
4	tablespoons	Brown sugar

Place all ingredients in a large bowl and mix. Marinate in refrigerator for at least 6 hours.

Place all ingredients in a baking pan and bake covered for 40 minutes and then 20 to 40 minutes uncovered until chicken is cooked and tender.

QUICK CHICKEN CREOLE

3 to 4 servings (VITAMIN K content of recipe without rice = 16 mcg per cup. The rice contains an insignificant amount of VITAMIN K when cooked.)

1	pound	Boneless, skinless chicken breast, cut into small chunks
14	ounces	Canned tomatoes plus juice
1	cup	Chopped green peppers
1/2	cup	Chopped celery
1/2	cup	Chopped onion
2	cloves	Minced garlic
1	teaspoon	Fresh basil, minced
1	teaspoon	Crushed red pepper
1/2	teaspoon	Salt
1/2	teaspoon	Chili powder
1	teaspoon	Olive or Canola oil, treated (See DIETARY TIP # 10.)

Cook chicken using the teaspoon of oil in hot skillet, turning often so that chicken is not burned. Cook chicken in this way until fully cooked. Remove chicken from pan and keep warm. Add remaining ingredients, bring to boil, then cook on low heat for 20 to 30 minutes. Add the chicken back to the pan. Heat. Best served on white rice.

CHICKEN GUMBO

4 to 6 servings (VITAMIN K content = 29 mcg per cup)

1 1/2	pounds	Skinless, boneless chicken pieces
3	cups	Water
1	teaspoon	Olive or Canola oil, treated (See DIETARY TIP # 10.)
1/4	cup	Flour
1	cup	Skinless potatoes, chopped
1	cup	Chopped onions
2	cups	Chopped carrots
1	cup	Chopped celery
4	cloves	Minced garlic
1/2	cup	Chopped scallion
1/2	teaspoon	Fresh thyme
1	teaspoon	Black pepper
1	cup	Sliced okra

Place oil and flour in large pot and heat mixture until flour is golden brown. Stir in the water. Add remainder of ingredients except okra and bring to a boil. Cook on low heat for 30 minutes. Add okra and cook on low heat for 15 more minutes or until okra is the desired tenderness.

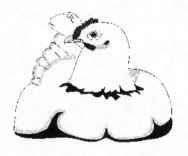

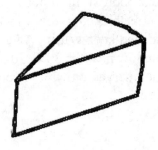

SAUCY HAM AND CHICKEN

8 servings (15 mcgs of VITAMIN K per serving.)

2		Broiler chickens, cut up
2	teaspoons	Oil, olive or Canola, treated (See DIETARY TIP # 10.)
1	cup	Fully cooked ham, in strips
2	medium	Onions, quartered (about 1 1/2 cups)
2	medium	Tomatoes (about 1 1/4 cups)
2	cups	CHEDDAR CHEESE SAUCE (See Recipe Index)
1	teaspoon	Fresh basil, minced

Season chicken with salt and pepper, brown on all sides in hot oil, drain. Transfer to crock pot.

Chop one tomato, combine with soup and basil, put ham in pot, pour sauce over meat.

Cover and cook on low 6-8 hours (or high 3-4 hours). Garnish with reserved tomato wedges and serve.

RASPBERRY CHICKEN BREASTS

4 servings (2 mcgs of VITAMIN K per serving.)

2		Whole chicken breast skinned (4 halves total about 5 ounces each)
2	tablespoons	Butter
1/4	cup	Raspberry jam, seedless
2	tablespoons	Balsamic vinegar

Sauté chicken breast in butter until just barely done. Slide chicken to the side of the skillet.

Add jam and vinegar, stir until jam is melted and mixed with vinegar, toss chicken in mixture to coat.

Serve chicken with sauce poured over the top.

LEMON ONION CHICKEN

4 to 6 servings (VITAMIN K content = less than 1 mcg per cup)

1 1/2	pounds	Boneless, skinless chicken
1/2	cup	Lemon juice
2	tablespoons	Vinegar
1/2	cup	Fresh minced lemon peel
1	teaspoon	Fresh minced oregano
3/4	cup	Chopped onion
1/2	teaspoon	Salt

Add all ingredients to baking dish and marinate for a few hours. Bake at 400 degrees Fahrenheit until the chicken is cooked. About 20 to 30 minutes depending on the thickness of the chicken pieces.

CHICKEN BREASTS DIANE
4 servings (24 mcgs of VITAMIN K per serving.)

8	3 ounce	Boneless chicken breast pieces (1 1/2 pounds)
1/2	teaspoon	Salt
2	tablespoons	Olive oil, treated (See DIETARY TIP # 10.)
1/2	teaspoon	Pepper
2	tablespoons	Butter
3	tablespoons	Fresh chives or green onions
		Juice of 1/2 lime or lemon
2	tablespoons	Brandy or cognac
2	teaspoons	Dijon-style mustard
1/4	cup	Chicken broth

Place chicken breast halves between sheets of waxed paper or plastic wrap. Pound slightly with mallet to even out the thickness of each piece. Sprinkle with salt and pepper.

Heat 1 tablespoon each of oil and butter in large skillet. Cook chicken over high heat for 2 minutes on each side. Do not cook longer or they will be overcooked and dry. Transfer to warm serving platter and keep warm.

Add chives or green onions, lime juice, brandy, and mustard to pan. Cook 15 seconds, whisking constantly. Whisk in broth. Stir until sauce is smooth. Whisk in remaining butter and oil. Pour sauce over chicken. Serve immediately.

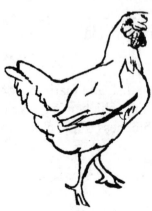

CHICKEN PICCATA

2 servings (1 mcgs of VITAMIN K per serving.)

1		Whole chicken breast, boned, skinned and flattened
		Salt and pepper
1 1/2	tablespoons	Flour
1/2	tablespoon	Olive oil, treated (See DIETARY TIP # 10.)
1	clove	Garlic, minced
1/4	pound	Mushrooms, sliced
1	teaspoon	Lemon juice
1/4	cup	Dry white wine

Dredge chicken in salt and pepper and flour.

In sauté pan over medium heat, melt butter with olive oil. Add garlic and sauté briefly. Add chicken breast and sauté for 1 - 2 minutes on each side and set aside.

Add mushrooms and sauté for 1 minute. Return chicken to pan and stir in lemon juice and wine and simmer covered for 10 minutes or until tender.

Put chicken on platter, spoon on juice and garnish with lemon.

TURKEY SPAGHETTI SAUCE

6 servings (20 mcgs of VITAMIN K per serving.)

1/4	cup	Onion, chopped
1	Clove	Garlic, minced
1	teaspoon	Olive oil, treated (See DIETARY TIP # 10.)
28	ounces	Canned tomatoes, cut up
6	ounces	Canned tomato paste
1	teaspoon	Basil, fresh chopped
1	teaspoon	Thyme, fresh chopped
3	cups	Cooked turkey, chopped
1	pound	Cooked noodles or pasta

Sauté the onion and garlic in the oil until lightly browned. Add the tomatoes, tomato paste, basil, thyme and turkey. Simmer for 20 to 25 minutes while cooking the noodles or pasta.

CHICKEN BREASTS WITH DRIED BEEF

8 servings (1 mcg of VITAMIN K per serving.)

8	4 ounce	Chicken breasts, boned, skinned and flattened
4	ounces	Dried beef
8		Bacon slices
1 1/2	cups	MUSHROOM CREAM SAUCE (See Recipe Index)
1/2	cup	White wine
1	cup	Sour cream
1/2	cup	Almonds, slivered

Place beef slices in chicken and roll up. Wrap bacon slices around chicken.

Place remaining slices of beef in 8x12x2 inch greased dish. Put chicken rolls on top of beef.

Mix sour cream, white wine and mushroom sauce. Pour over chicken.

Bake at 350 degrees Fahrenheit for 1 hour uncovered. After the first 30 minutes, sprinkle the almonds on top. Finish baking.

Serve with rice, noodles or mashed potatoes.

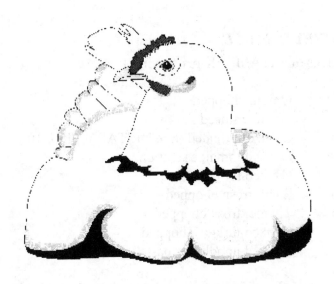

MARSALA CHICKEN BREASTS

8 servings (Less than 1 mcg of VITAMIN K per serving.)

8	3 ounce	Chicken breasts, de-boned
		Salt and pepper
2	tablespoons	Butter
1	tablespoon	Canola or Olive oil, treated (See DIETARY TIP # 10.)
1	pound	Mushrooms, halved
2	tablespoons	Flour
3/4	cup	Marsala wine
1/2	cup	Chicken broth
1	clove	Garlic, minced
1		Lemon, sliced for garnish

Salt and pepper chicken breasts.

Melt butter in a skillet and add oil.

Sauté chicken breasts on both sides, until browned. Remove to a platter.

Add mushrooms to the skillet and sauté for 2 minutes. Sprinkle with the flour, blending well.

Add the wine to the skillet. Stir up any browned bits on the pan into the wine. Add garlic and chicken broth. Heat until thickened.

Cut chicken into bite size pieces, return to skillet and toss with ingredients. Turn onto a serving platter and garnish with lemon slices.

This is also excellent with veal.

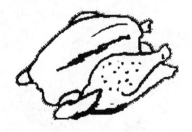

SAUTÉ CHICKEN BREAST WITH MUSHROOMS

2 servings (2 mcgs of VITAMIN K per serving.)

2	4 ounce	Chicken breasts, boneless
1	cup	Fresh mushrooms, quartered
4	tablespoons	Clarified butter
		Flour for dredging
		Salt and pepper to taste
1	cup	Water
1/2		Lemon, juice only

Pound chicken breasts thin. Dredge in flour and shake off excess.

In a large skillet, pour in the butter and put in the chicken breasts. Brown lightly on both sides.

Add mushrooms, lemon juice, salt, pepper and toss.

Add water, reduce over high heat until sauce thickens slightly.

Remove breasts, place on warmed serving plate. Spoon sauce and mushrooms over chicken, garnish with a twist of lemon.

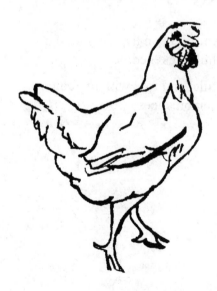

CHICKEN SAUTÉ BOURGUIGNONNE

6 servings (2 mcgs of VITAMIN K per serving.)

3	pounds	Chicken breasts, split in half, boneless, skinless
		Salt and pepper to taste
4	tablespoons	Butter
1/2	pound	Fresh mushrooms, trimmed and sliced
1/2	cup	Onion, chopped
1		Bay leaf
1	clove	Garlic, chopped
1/2	teaspoon	Fresh thyme
1	tablespoon	Flour
1/2	cup	Chicken broth
1	cup	Burgundy wine or other dry red wine

Flatten chicken breasts between waxed paper to 1/4 inch thickness. Season with salt and pepper to taste. Cut each cutlet into quarters.

Heat 2 tablespoon butter in large heavy skillet. Cook chicken 5 minutes or until no longer pink in center, turning over halfway through cooking. Transfer chicken to a platter.

Add mushrooms to skillet, cook 2 minutes. Add onion, shallot, bay leaf, garlic and thyme, cook, stirring, for 1 minute. Sprinkle with flour, stirring to blend. Stir in broth and wine. Simmer 2 minutes. Whisk in remaining butter to thicken slightly.

Add chicken, heat through. Season with salt and pepper. Remove bay leaf. Serve chicken with sauce spooned over top.

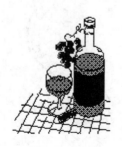

ROAST TURKEY

12 servings (2 mcgs of VITAMIN K per serving.)

1	12 pound	Turkey
1	tablespoon	Canola oil, treated (See DIETARY TIP # 10.)
		Black pepper, ground
1	medium	Onion, peeled
1		Bay leaf
1	teaspoon	Thyme, fresh

Preheat oven to 350 degrees Fahrenheit.

Sprinkle the turkey, inside and out, with pepper. Put the bay leaf and thyme inside the cavity.

Rub the turkey all over with oil. Put the turkey, breast side up, in a roasting pan and arrange the onion, neck and gizzard around it.

Bake for 1 hour and cover loosely with a sheet of aluminum foil. Continue baking, basting at 10-minute intervals, for about 1 1/2 hours longer.

Transfer the turkey to a platter and pour off the pan drippings into a strainer and remove fat. Serve with the natural juices.

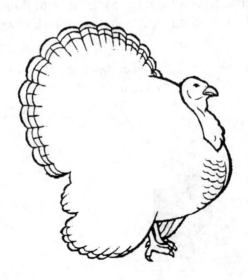

LAMB

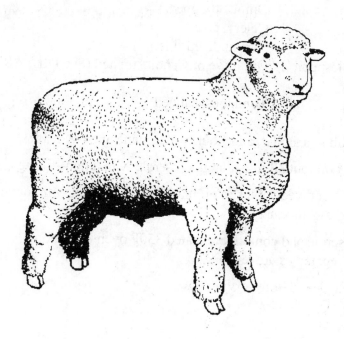

OVEN-COOKED LAMB STEW

6 servings (5 mcg of VITAMIN K per serving.)

3	pounds	Lamb stew meat,1 1/2 inch cubes
3	tablespoons	Flour
1 1/2	cups	Water
1 1/4	cups	Red wine
		Salt to taste
		Pepper to taste
1		Bay leaf
1	clove	Garlic, minced
3/4	cup	Onion, chopped
1/2	cup	Celery, coarse, diced
1/2	cup	Carrot, diced fine
1	tablespoon	Oil, olive or Canola, treated (See DIETARY TIP # 10.)
1	cup	Tomatoes, canned

Brown lamb in a skillet, add flour, water, wine and bay leaf.

Bring to a boil, put all into a large casserole with a tight-fitting cover.

Sauté garlic and vegetables in oil until limp, add them with tomatoes to the lamb and gravy mixture.

Cover casserole and cook in preheated 350F oven 1 1/2 hours, or until lamb and vegetables are tender.

Remove bay leaf before serving.

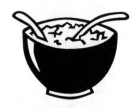

GREEK-ROAST LEG OF LAMB

5 servings (Less than 2 mcg of VITAMIN K per serving.)

6	pounds	Lamb leg
1/2	cup	Olive oil, treated (See DIETARY TIP # 10.)
3	cloves	Garlic, crushed
1	teaspoon	Oregano, fresh minced
		Black pepper, freshly ground
		Salt

For rare lamb, allow the lamb to come to room temperature. Heat your oven to 400 degrees Fahrenheit.

Mix the oil, garlic and oregano together and rub the leg completely with the mixture. Season with salt and black pepper and place on a baking rack in a pan. Insert a meat thermometer in the thickest part of the leg, being careful not to touch the bone.

Bake at 400 degrees Fahrenheit for 40 minutes so the meat can brown. Turn the oven down to 325 degrees Fahrenheit and bake for an additional 40 to 50 minutes, or until the thermometer registers 140 degrees Fahrenheit.

Remove the meat from the oven and allow it to sit 1/2 hour before slicing. It will continue to cook during this time.

For medium lamb: Follow the above instructions but cook a bit longer so that the thermometer registers 145 to 150 degrees Fahrenheit.

Slice thin and serve with some of the pan juices.

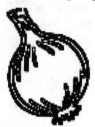

LEG OF LAMB

8 servings (2 mcgs of VITAMIN K per serving.)

8	pounds	Leg of lamb
2	cloves	Garlic, slivered
1/2	cup	Butter
1/2	teaspoon	Fresh rosemary
1/2		Lemon, juice only
12		Pearl onions
		Salt and pepper

Wash and dry the lamb. Make incisions and stuff with slivers of garlic. Place in roasting pan.

Melt butter in a saucepan, add rosemary and the lemon juice and spread the mixture over the lamb in the roasting pan.

Bake at 325 degrees Fahrenheit for 2-1/2 to 3 hours. Serve with rice and vegetables.

CROWN ROAST OF LAMB

6 to 8 servings (Less than 1 mcg of VITAMIN K per serving.)

1		Crown roast of lamb (2 or more ribs per person, depending on size)
3	cloves	Garlic peeled and cut in slivers
1/4	cup	Olive oil, treated (See DIETARY TIP # 10.)
2	teaspoons	Freshly ground pepper
12		New potatoes, peeled (allow 2-to-3 for each diner)
1	tablespoon	Salt

Preheat oven to 450 degrees Fahrenheit.

Make small incisions in the meaty part of the lamb every few inches and insert slivers of garlic. Paint the meat well with olive oil. Sprinkle all over with pepper. Crumple a ball of aluminum foil and stuff in the center.

Place on a small rack and surround with the potatoes in a low roasting pan just large enough to hold it.

Place in the oven and immediately turn the heat down to 400 degrees Fahrenheit. Roast until done, depending upon weight and size, about 30 minutes or until internal temperature reaches 140 degrees Fahrenheit.

Remove the foil ball and immediately salt the meat. Remove to a warmed platter, and let rest 5-to-10 minutes before serving. If waiting longer, cover with foil to retain heat.

To serve, place paper frills on the rib bones and fill the center with vegetables or stuffing, surround with potatoes and garnish with watercress or curly endive. (Do not eat the watercress or endive. The VITAMIN K content is too high. Garnish only.) Any sauce would be served on the side.

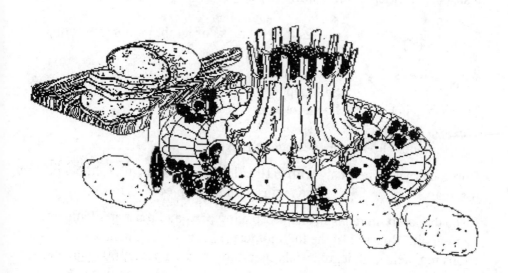

MUSTARD & WINE MARINATED LAMB CHOPS

4 servings (1 mcg of VITAMIN K per serving.)

4		Sirloin lamb chops 1 inch thick
1	teaspoon	Salt
3	tablespoons	Stone ground mustard
1/4	teaspoon	pepper
1	cup	Red wine

Rub both sides of chops with mustard. Sprinkle with salt and pepper. Cover with wine and marinate overnight in refrigerator.

Rub again with mustard just before broiling or pan-frying to desired doneness.

ARTILLERY RACK OF LAMB

8 servings (1 mcg of VITAMIN K per serving.)

2	racks	(3 1/2- to 4-lb) racks of lamb, with 8 to 9 chops each
2 to 3	cloves	Garlic, split
		Salt, pepper
1/2	teaspoon	Fresh rosemary, crushed

Have butcher "French" bone ends of racks.

Rub each rack generously with garlic. Lightly season with salt, pepper and rosemary. Cover exposed bone tips with small pieces of foil.

Place the lamb on racks in shallow baking pans and roast at 375 degrees Fahrenheit. Roast until the thermometer placed in the thickest part of the chops registers 140 degrees Fahrenheit for medium rare, 160 degrees Fahrenheit for medium or 170 degrees Fahrenheit for well done. Remove roasts from oven and place bone sides together, intertwining ends of rib bones to resemble stacked rifles.

Discard foil and cover bone tips with paper frills, if desired.

Allow to stand 10 minutes before carving.

ATHENIAN LAMB STEW

4 servings (16 mcgs of VITAMIN K per serving.)

3/4	cup	Onion, minced
1	clove	Garlic, crushed
1	tablespoon	Chopped, fresh basil
2	pounds	Lean lamb shoulder or leg, cubed
3	tablespoons	Olive oil, treated (See DIETARY TIP # 10.)
		Salt, pepper
28	ounces	Whole tomatoes, crushed
1/2	cup	Rose wine
1	cup	Cut carrots
3	medium	Potatoes, peeled and quartered
1	2 inch stick	Cinnamon

Sauté onion, garlic and basil with lamb in oil until onion is tender. Season to taste with salt and pepper. Continue cooking until lamb is lightly browned.

Add crushed tomatoes and wine. Cook 10 minutes.

Add carrots, potatoes and cinnamon stick. Cover and cook over low heat 1 to 1 1/2 hours, or until lamb is very tender.

Serve with rice or noodles.

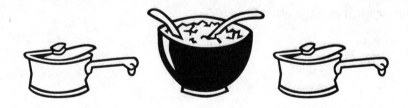

GRILLED LAMB AND SAUSAGE KEBABS
6 servings (4 mcg of VITAMIN K per serving.)

1	pound	Lamb boneless shoulder, cut into 1-inch cubes
1/2	cup	Olive oil, treated (See DIETARY TIP # 10.)
3	tablespoons	Lemon juice
1/2	teaspoon	Salt
1/2	teaspoon	Pepper
1	clove	Garlic
1	pound	Sweet Italian sausage links
18		Bay leaves
18		Fresh mushroom caps

Place lamb in glass or plastic bowl. Process oil, lemon juice, salt, pepper and garlic in food processor or blender until smooth. Pour over lamb. Cover and refrigerate 30 minutes. Remove lamb from marinade. Reserve marinade.

Cut sausage into eighteen 1-inch pieces. Alternate lamb, sausage, bay leaves and mushroom caps on each of six 10-inch metal skewers, leaving space between each piece of food. Cover and grill kebabs (about 4 inches from hot coals) 10 minutes, turning kebabs and brushing with marinade occasionally, until meat is done. (Do not eat the bay leaves.)

NOTE: To broil, place kebabs on rack in broiler pan. Broil with tops about 3 inches from heat 5 minutes. Turn kebabs. Brush with marinade. Broil 5 minutes. Turn kebabs. Brush with marinade. Broil 5 minutes longer or until meat is done.

PORK

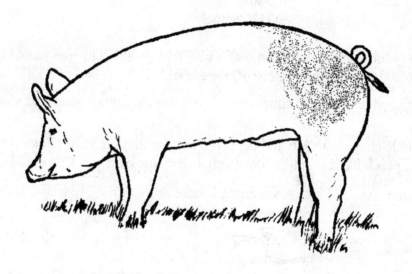

PEACHY PORK CHOPS

6 servings (8 mcgs of VITAMIN K per serving.)

6	4 ounce	Pork chops
1/4	cup	Brown sugar, plus 1 tablespoon
1/2	teaspoon	Cinnamon
1/4	teaspoon	Cloves
8	ounces	Tomato sauce
4	cups	Peaches, fresh, peeled, pit removed
1/4	cup	Water
1/4	cup	Vinegar
		Salt and pepper

Lightly brown pork chops on both sides in large skillet or slow-cooking pot with browning unit. Pour off excess fat.

Combine brown sugar, cinnamon, cloves, tomato sauce, water and vinegar.

Sprinkle chops with salt and pepper. Arrange chops in slow cooking pot. Place peach halves on top. Pour tomato mixture over all. Cover and cook on low for 4 to 6 hours.

PORK CHOPS BRAISED WITH CIDER AND APPLES

4 servings (1 mcg of VITAMIN K per serving.)

4		Pork chops 3/4 inch thick
1	tablespoon	Oil, olive or Canola, treated (See DIETARY TIP # 10.)
2	tablespoons	Butter, 1/4 stick
1	cup	Onion, thinly sliced
1/2	cup	Apple, tart, peeled
1/2	cup	Apple cider
1 1/2	tablespoons	Apple cider vinegar
1		Bay leaf

Season pork chops generously with salt and pepper. Heat oil in heavy large skillet over medium-high heat. Add pork to skillet and cook until brown and cooked through, about 10 to 15 minutes per side. Transfer pork to platter. Tent with foil to keep warm.

Drain off all but 1 tablespoon drippings from skillet. Add butter to skillet and melt over medium heat. Add onion and peeled apple to skillet and sauté until onion is almost soft, about 5 minutes. Mix in cider, vinegar and bay leaf. Cover skillet and cook until onions and apples are tender, about 10 minutes.

Discard bay leaf. Add any accumulated juices from pork chop platter to skillet. Increase heat and cook until sauce thickens slightly, about three minutes. Spoon sauce over pork chops and serve.

NEAPOLITAN PORK CHOPS

6 servings (6 mcgs of VITAMIN K per serving.)

2	tablespoons	Oil, olive or Canola, treated
1	clove	Garlic
6		Pork chops
		Salt and pepper
3	tablespoons	Tomato paste
3	tablespoons	Water
3/4	cup	Green pepper, chopped
1	cup	Mushrooms, sliced

In a skillet, heat oil and add garlic and cook until browned. Discard garlic. Add chops and brown. Salt and pepper, and add remaining ingredients. Cover and simmer over low heat 30 to 35 minutes.

BAKED PORK CHOPS

6 to 8 servings (The pork itself contains little vitamin k. The mixture on top of the pork chops contains 20 micrograms of VITAMIN K per cup. If you do not use green peppers, this recipe contains almost no VITAMIN K.)

3	pounds	Lean pork chops
1	cup	Onions, finely chopped
1	cup	Green peppers
1/4	teaspoon	Black pepper
1/4	teaspoon	Salt

Remove fat from pork chops and place in baking pan. Mix all other ingredients together and spread on chops. Bake at 350 degrees Fahrenheit until pork chops are cooked, approximately 30 to 40 minutes.

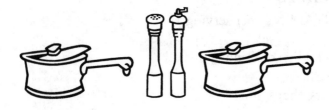

GLAZED PORK LOIN ROAST

8 servings (2 mcgs of VITAMIN K per serving.)

1		Fresh pork loin roast, boneless (2 1/2 pounds)
1	clove	Garlic, cut into slivers
1	teaspoon	Salt
1	tablespoon	Orange marmalade
1	teaspoon	Prepared mustard
1	teaspoon	Fresh thyme leaves

Preheat oven to 350 degrees Fahrenheit.

Make slits in the fat on the pork roast with the tip of a sharp knife. Insert a piece of garlic in each slit. Sprinkle roast with salt.

Mix marmalade, mustard and thyme together and spread on the roast. Place roast in roasting pan. Cover pan with lid or foil. Place in oven and roast for 1 1/2 hours or until roast registers 170 degrees Fahrenheit on a meat thermometer.

Serve with meat juices.

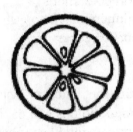

LEMON PECAN PORK CHOPS

4 servings (1 mcg of VITAMIN K per serving.)

4		Boneless pork loin chops
2	tablespoons	Finely chopped pecans
1/2	teaspoon	Garlic salt
3	tablespoons	Fresh lemon juice
1/4	teaspoon	Lemon pepper seasoning
1	tablespoon	Butter or Canola oil, treated (See DIETARY TIP # 10.)
		Fresh lemon slices optional

Sprinkle both sides of chops with garlic salt and lemon pepper.

Heat butter or oil in large skillet over medium heat. Add chops and brown 5 to 7 minutes per side or until pork is tender. Remove chops to a serving plate, sprinkle with pecans and keep warm.

Stir lemon juice into drippings in skillet, heat for one minute, stirring constantly. Spoon over cooked chops. Garnish with lemon slices.

PORK PINWHEELS WITH APRICOT STUFFING

4 servings (5 mcgs of VITAMIN K per serving.)

1	pound	Pork tenderloin

SAUCE

1 1/2	teaspoon	Cornstarch
		Nutmeg (dash)
1	cup	Apricot nectar

APRICOT STUFFING

1	teaspoon	Bouillon, chicken, instant granules
2/3	cup	Water, hot
1/3	cup	Apricots, dried, snipped
2	tablespoons	Celery, chopped
1	tablespoon	Butter
1/8	teaspoon	Cinnamon, ground
		Pepper, black, (dash)
2	cups	Bread cubes

Split tenderloin lengthwise, cutting to, but not through, opposite side, open out flat. Pound tenderloin lightly with meat mallet to a 10x6 rectangle.

APRICOT STUFFING - Dissolve bouillon in hot water and pour over apricots. Let stand 5 minutes. Cook celery and onion in butter until tender but not brown. Remove from heat and stir in cinnamon and pepper. In a large bowl, mix the bread cubes, onion mixture, and apricot mixture and toss lightly to moisten.

Spread stuffing evenly over tenderloin. Roll up jelly-roll style, starting from short side. Secure meat roll with wooden toothpicks or tie with string at 1-inch intervals. Cut meat roll into six 1-inch slices. Place meat slices on rack of unheated broiler pan, cut side down. Broil 4 inches from heat 12 minutes. Turn, broil 11 to 13 minutes more or until done. Remove toothpicks or string, transfer meat to a serving platter.

Meanwhile, for SAUCE, combine cornstarch and nutmeg. Stir in apricot nectar. Cook and stir until mixture is bubbly. Cook and stir 2 minutes more.

SERVE sauce with meat slices.

BAKED HAM WITH PINEAPPLE

12 servings (Less than 1 mcg of VITAMIN K per serving.)

2	pounds	Smoked ham, fully cooked, boneless
20		Cloves, whole
4	slices	Pineapple, unsweetened, canned, drained
1/2	cup	Ginger ale, diet or regular
1	teaspoon	Ground cinnamon

Remove and discard casing from ham. Score top of ham in a diamond design, and stud with cloves.

Place ham in shallow baking dish, and arrange pineapple slices over top. Pour ginger ale over ham, and sprinkle each pineapple slice with cinnamon.

Bake ham at 325 degrees Fahrenheit for 45 to 60 minutes until thoroughly heated.

Cut into 12 slices and serve.

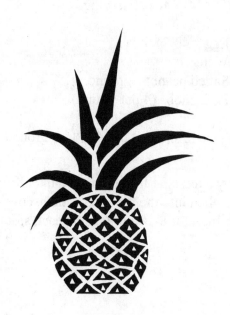

GRILLED BRATWURST

6 servings (Less than 1 mcg of VITAMIN K per serving.)

6		Bratwursts, (1 1/2 pounds)
12	ounces	Beer
1	medium	Onion, chopped
6		Peppercorns
4	whole	Cloves
6		Hard rolls

Place Bratwursts, beer, onion, peppercorns, and cloves in a 3-quart saucepan. Simmer for 20 minutes. Drain.

Grill Bratwursts 2 to 5 inches from charcoal about 10 minutes, until browned. Sprinkle with water to form a crisp skin.

Serve in hard rolls with mustard.

PEANUT PORK CHOPS

4 servings (1 mcg of VITAMIN K per serving.)

1	large	Egg
1/4	cup	Water
1/2	cup	Salted peanuts, ground
4	lean	Pork chops (4 per pound)

Beat egg with water. Place in shallow bowl. Place ground peanuts in another shallow bowl.

Remove and discard any excess fat from chops. Dip chops first into the egg, shaking off excess, then into the ground peanuts, covering each chop. Grill chops on medium-high for 8-10 minutes on each side.

PORK CHOPS WITH ONIONS

4 servings (Less than 1 mcg of VITAMIN K per serving.)

4		Pork chops
1/2	teaspoon	Salt
1/4	teaspoon	Pepper
1 1/2	tablespoons	Flour
1 1/2	tablespoons	Oil, olive or Canola, treated (See DIETARY TIP # 10.)
2	medium	Onions, thinly sliced
1/2	cup	Beer
1/2	cup	Beef broth, hot
1	teaspoon	Cornstarch

Season pork chops with salt and pepper and coat with flour.

Heat oil in a heavy frying pan. Add pork chops, fry for 3 minutes on each side.

Add onions, cook for another 5 minutes, turning chops once.

Pour in beer and beef broth, cover and simmer 15 minutes.

Remove pork shops to a preheated platter.

Blend cornstarch with a small amount of cold water. Stir into sauce and cook until thick and bubbly.

Pour over pork chops.

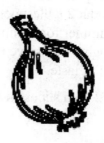

GRILLED PORK TENDERLOIN WITH MUSTARD CREAM

4 servings (Less than 1 mcg of VITAMIN K per serving.)

1 1/2	pounds	Pork tenderloin, trimmed
3/4	cup	Oil, Canola or olive, treated (See DIETARY TIP # 10.)
3/4	cup	Dry white wine

SAUCE

1/4	cup	Dry white wine
3	cloves	Garlic, crushed
3/4	cup	Dry white wine
1	tablespoon	Shallots, minced
1	cup	Heavy cream
3	tablespoons	Dijon-style mustard
1	dash	White pepper

In a small deep dish just large enough to hold the pork, combine the oil, 3/4 cup wine and garlic. Add the pork, turning it to coat thoroughly and let it marinate, covered and chilled, overnight.

Drain the pork and discard the marinade. Grill the pork on an oiled rack set about 6 inches over glowing coals. Turn it for 25 minutes, or until a meat thermometer registers 155 degrees Fahrenheit, for meat that is just cooked through but still juicy.

Transfer the pork to a cutting board and let it stand while making the sauce.

SAUCE: In a small heavy saucepan, boil 1/4 cup white wine with the shallots until it is reduced to about 2 tablespoons. Add the cream, bring the mixture just to a boil and simmer for 2 minutes, or until it is thickened slightly. Strain the sauce through a fine sieve into a bowl and whisk in the mustard, white pepper, and salt to taste.

Cut the pork diagonally into 1/2 inch slices and serve it with the mustard cream sauce.

MUSHROOM SAUSAGE PIE

6 servings (5 mcgs of VITAMIN K per serving.)

1	9 inch	Pie shell, single crust
1	pound	Hot pork sausage
1/4	cup	Butter
12	ounces	Fresh mushrooms
1	cup	Whipping cream, not whipped
2		Egg yolks, beaten
1	tablespoon	Flour
1	tablespoon	Melted butter
1	tablespoon	Lemon juice
1/2	teaspoon	Salt
1/2	teaspoon	Pepper
1/2	cup	Freshly grated Parmesan cheese

Preheat oven to 450 degrees Fahrenheit.

Roll out and fit pastry into 9-inch pie plate. Without pricking, bake the crust about 8 to 10 minutes, until lightly brown. As it bakes, air pockets underneath the pastry can cause it to puff up and crack. So check the pastry every 2 or 3 minutes and push it down to fit the shape of the pie plate if this happens. Let stand while making filling.

In a large skillet, fry the pork sausage and drain fat well. In the same skillet, melt the butter, add mushrooms, and cook briefly. Spread the sausage and mushrooms evenly in the pastry.

In a medium mixing bowl, whisk together thoroughly the heavy cream, egg yolks, flour, melted butter, lemon juice, salt, and pepper. Pour this mixture evenly over the pie filling. Bake the pie for 30 or 40 minutes at 375 degrees Fahrenheit, until rich brown and set. As you remove from the oven, sprinkle the Parmesan cheese over the top. Serve warm.

HAM IN ZIPPY CREAM SAUCE

4 servings (1 mcg of VITAMIN K per serving.)

| 1 | pound | Smoked ham, in cubes |

CREAM SAUCE

3	tablespoons	Flour
3	tablespoons	Butter
1 1/2	cups	Milk
1	teaspoon	Dijon mustard
1	teaspoon	Horseradish, fresh

Sauté ham cubes until lightly browned.

Melt butter in sauce pan, add flour and mix thoroughly. Add milk and stir continuously until sauce thickens and comes to just bubbling. Add mustard and horseradish, stir and allow to heat through. Add ham cubes and allow to heat through.

To serve over noodles, add more milk to make the sauce thinner.

HAM AND CHEESE PIE

6 servings (21 mcgs of VITAMIN K per serving.)

12	ounces	Creamed cottage cheese, drained
3	ounces	Cream cheese, softened
1	cup	Shredded cheddar cheese (4 ounces)
2	large	Eggs
1	cup	Cut-up cooked smoked ham
1	cup	Bisquick (low-fat) or similar baking mix
1/4	cup	Milk
2	large	Eggs
1/4	cup	Sliced green onions
1	tablespoon	Toasted sesame seed

Heat oven to 375 degrees Fahrenheit. Lightly grease a 9 inch pie plate.

Mix cheeses, 2 eggs and the ham, reserve. Mix Bisquick, milk, 2 eggs and onions together. Beat vigorously for about 20 strokes.

Spread half of the batter in pie plate. Spoon reserved cheese mixture evenly over batter in pie plate. Carefully spread remaining batter over cheese mixture. Sprinkle with sesame seed.

Bake until knife inserted halfway between center and edge comes out clean, 35 to 40 minutes. Let stand 5 minutes before cutting.

PORK LOIN WITH MUSTARD CRUST

4 servings (9 mcgs of VITAMIN K per serving.)

2	pounds	Pork loin or tenderloin
		Salt to taste
		Fresh ground pepper to taste
1 1/2	cups	Bread crumbs, home made, if possible
1	tablespoons	Chopped fresh basil
1		Shallot
1	clove	Garlic
1/2	cup	Grainy mustard

Trim away any fat and season pork loin with salt and pepper.

Lightly toast bread crumbs in 400 degree Fahrenheit oven but do not let them brown too much. (You can toast them at a lower heat, it will just take longer.)

Mince herbs, shallot and garlic and stir into bread crumbs.

Using pastry brush, paint pork all over with mustard and then dredge in crumb mixture. Place loin in oiled roasting pan. Bake at 400 degrees Fahrenheit 30 minutes, or until internal temperature reaches 150 degrees Fahrenheit. Let roast stand 5 minutes before carving. Cut into 1/2 inch slices and serve at once.

PORK CHOPS PARMESAN

4 servings (3 mcg of VITAMIN K per serving.)

3	tablespoons	Cornmeal, whole-wheat flour, or bread crumbs
1	tablespoon	Parmesan cheese, grated
1/2	teaspoon	Pepper, black
1/2	teaspoon	Salt,
1/2	teaspoon	Basil, fresh chopped
4		Pork loin rib chops, about 1/2-inch thick
1	tablespoon	Oil, olive or Canola, treated (See DIETARY TIP # 10.)
1/2	cup	Onions, chopped
1	clove	Garlic, minced
1/4	teaspoon	Fennel seeds, crushed

Combine the cornmeal, Parmesan cheese, black pepper, salt, and basil.

Trim the pork chops of all visible fat, pat them dry, and dredge in the cornmeal mixture.

Heat a skillet over medium heat, and add the oil. When the oil is hot, place the chops in the skillet and reduce the heat to low. Fry the chops for 10 minutes on each side. Then add the onions, garlic, fennel, and continue frying for another 10 minutes, turning as necessary to keep from sticking.

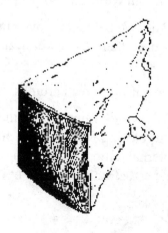

PORK MARENGO

6 servings (8 mcg of VITAMIN K per serving.)

2	pounds	Pork shoulder, boneless, cut in 1 inch cubes
1/2	cup	Onion, chopped
2	tablespoons	Oil, Canola or olive, treated (See DIETARY TIP # 10.)
16	ounces	Tomatoes, cut up
1	teaspoon	Chicken bouillon granules
1	teaspoon	Marjoram, fresh, minced
1	teaspoon	Salt
1	teaspoon	Thyme, fresh, minced
	dash	Pepper
3	ounces	Mushrooms, canned, chopped and drained
1/3	cup	Water
3	tablespoons	Flour, all purpose
		Rice

In skillet, brown half of the pork cubes and chopped onion, (at a time) in the hot oil. Drain off fat. Transfer meat and onion to a crock pot.

In the same skillet combine undrained tomatoes, bouillon granules, marjoram, salt, thyme and pepper. Stir together, scraping browned bits from bottom of skillet. Pour over pork.

Cover, cook on LOW for 4 to 6 hours. Turn to HIGH. Stir in drained mushrooms.

Blend cold water slowly into flour and stir into the pork mixture. Cook, uncovered, on HIGH until thickened, 15 to 20 minutes, stirring occasionally.

Serve over rice or noodles.

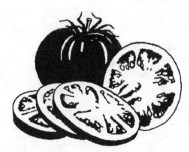

PORK CHOPS IN TOMATO SAUCE WITH OREGANO

4 servings (20 mcgs of VITAMIN K per serving.)

2	cups	Plum tomatoes, diced
1/4	cup	Water
		Salt and pepper
4		Loin pork chops
2	tablespoons	Olive oil, treated (See DIETARY TIP # 10.)
2	teaspoons	Garlic, chopped
1 1/2	cups	Mushrooms, thin sliced
1 1/2	cups	Green pepper, cut in 1 inch cubes
1/2	cup	Dry white wine
1	teaspoon	Fresh oregano

Put the tomatoes with the water and bring to a boil, stirring occasionally.

Sprinkle the chops with salt and pepper.

Heat the oil in the skillet and add the chops. Brown on both sides, about 5 minutes to a side. Add the garlic and mushrooms.

Stir in the wine, tomatoes and oregano. Cover closely and cook 35 to 40 minutes.

Serve with pasta.

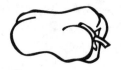

SEAFOOD

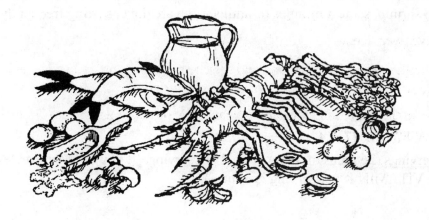

SAUTÉED GARLIC SHRIMP

2 servings (1 mcg of VITAMIN K per serving.)

3	cloves	Garlic minced
1/4	cup	Butter
3	tablespoons	Fresh lemon juice
2	tablespoons	Dry vermouth
2	teaspoons	Wine vinegar
		Dash of salt
2	Drops	Tabasco
1	pound	Shrimp, peeled, deveined and drained
		Hot cooked rice

Sauté garlic in butter in a skillet.

Combine the next 7 ingredients, and slowly add this mixture to the skillet, add shrimp, sauté 5 minutes or until shrimp are done, stirring frequently.

Serve over rice.

PAN FRIED TUNA

4 servings (26 mcgs of VITAMIN K per serving. If you omit the parsley, the VITAMIN K per serving is 3 mcg.)

4	6 ounce	Tuna steaks
1/2	cup	Flour, all purpose
1/2	cup	Olive oil, treated (See DIETARY TIP # 10.)
1	cup	Onion, thinly sliced
1/4	cup	Chicken stock
1 1/2	tablespoons	White wine vinegar
1	tablespoon	Parsley, fresh, chopped
		Black pepper, freshly ground
		Salt

Roll the tuna steaks in flour and pat off the excess.

Heat a large frying pan and add the oil. Pan-fry the fish over medium heat, about 1 to 2 minutes per side, and remove to a warm plate. Do not overcook.

Discard half the oil and return the pan to the heat. Add the onion, chicken stock, vinegar, and black pepper to taste. Sauté for about 5 minutes until the onion just becomes tender and the sauce reduces a bit. Add the parsley and salt to taste. Spoon the sauce over the warm fish and serve.

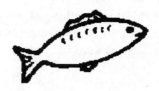

PEPPER GRILLED SALMON
4 servings (2 mcgs of VITAMIN K per serving.)

1	pound	Salmon fillets
1	teaspoon	Black peppercorns
1	teaspoon	Anise seeds
1/2	teaspoon	Coarse (kosher) salt
		Olive or Canola oil for grill rack

Coat grill rack with oil. Place grill rack 5 inch from coals.

In a clean coffee grinder or spice mill, grind peppercorns, anise seeds and salt until coarsely ground. Sprinkle over salmon.

Grill salmon 4 to 5 minutes on each side or until cooked through. Serve hot.

BAKED FISH

4 servings (VITAMIN K content = 10 mcg per cup of mixture on top of fish. Add 5 mcg VITAMIN K for every 100 grams of fish ONLY if mackerel is used.)

This recipe can be used with any of the types of fish we know have a very low amount of VITAMIN K. These include butterfly bream, eel, mackerel, salmon, tuna, and yellowtail (snapper). It is very likely that many other fish will be added to this list when more data regarding the VITAMIN K content of various fish species is determined. However, for now, the above list is all we have.

Also, since the above fish contains little VITAMIN K, the amount of fish that you use in this recipe will not significantly change VITAMIN K intake. The only possible exception to this is mackerel, which contains 5 mcg of VITAMIN K per 100 grams or about 22 1/2 mcg of VITAMIN K per pound.

4	portions	Fish
3	tablespoons	Lime or lemon juice
1/2	cup	Finely chopped onion
1	cup	Finely chopped tomatoes
1/2	teaspoon	Olive or Canola oil, treated (See DIETARY TIP # 10.)
1/2	teaspoon	Black pepper
1/4	teaspoon	Salt

Place fish in baking dish. Mix above ingredients and pour over fish. Bake at 350 degrees Fahrenheit until fish is cooked (usually 10 to 20 minutes).

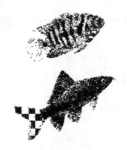

MEDITERRANEAN BAKED FISH

4 servings (VITAMIN K content of SAUCE ONLY = 7 mcg per cup)

This recipe can be used with any of the types of fish we know have a very low amount of VITAMIN K. These include butterfly bream, eel, mackerel, salmon, tuna, and yellowtail (snapper). However, it will probably taste best with bream, tuna, or yellowtail. It is very likely that other fish will be added to this list when more data regarding the VITAMIN K content of various fish species is determined. Also, since the above fish contains little VITAMIN K, the amount of fish you use in this recipe will not significantly change the VITAMIN K intake. The only possible exception to this is mackerel, which contains 5 mcg of VITAMIN K per 100 grams or about 22 1/2 mcgs of VITAMIN K per pound.

2	teaspoons	Olive oil, treated (See DIETARY TIP # 10.)
1	cup	Sliced or diced onions
2	cups	Whole chopped tomatoes, plus juice
1	clove	Minced garlic
1	cup	White wine
1/2	cup	Lemon or lime juice
1/2	teaspoon	Fresh chopped oregano
1/4	teaspoon	Black pepper

Sauté onion and garlic in olive oil. Add all remaining ingredients and cook on low heat for 30 minutes to make sauce. Cover approximately 1 pound of fish with sauce and bake until fish cooked.

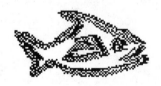

ARTICHOKE BOTTOMS WITH SHRIMP SAUTÉ

6 servings (9 mcgs of VITAMIN K per serving.)

6		Artichoke bottoms, frozen (approximately 1 cup)
1	quart	Water
1	tablespoon	Salt
3	ounces	Butter
1	tablespoon	Onion, minced
1	clove	Garlic, minced
1	tablespoon	Bell pepper, minced
1	tablespoon	Pimento, minced
1/4	pound	Fresh mushrooms, sliced
1/4	teaspoon	Thyme, fresh
1/2	teaspoon	Dill weed, fresh
1 1/2	pounds	Shrimp, peeled, deveined and chopped
		Salt and pepper

Bring the salted water to a boil and add the artichoke bottoms. Cook for 5 minutes or until tender. Drain and keep warm.

Melt the butter in a skillet and add the onion, garlic, bell pepper and pimento. Cook over moderate heat for 5 minutes and add the mushrooms, thyme and dill weed. Sauté for 3 minutes and add the shrimp. Toss for 4 minutes over high heat. Correct the seasonings and spoon over artichokes.

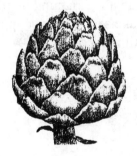

SALMON GRILL DIABLE

6 servings (1 mcg of VITAMIN K per serving.)

1/3	cup	Butter, soft
2	tablespoons	Lemon juice
2	teaspoons	Dijon mustard
6	large	Salmon steaks or fillets, 1 inch thick, 4 to 5 ounces each
		Olive oil, treated (See DIETARY TIP # 10.)
		Salt and pepper

Beat the butter until creamy, gradually adding lemon juice until mixture is fluffy. Beat in mustard. (Cover and chill if you are making it ahead.)

Bring butter mixture to room temperature. Lightly coat salmon steaks with olive oil, using pastry brush. Sprinkle with salt and pepper. Set salmon on grill 6 inch above hot gray coals. Cook, turning once with wide spatula, until fish flakes in center when prodded with fork, about 10 minutes.

Place steaks on hot serving platter, topping each with equal portion of butter mixture.

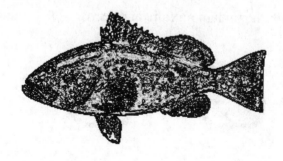

SHRIMP WITH TOMATO SAUCE

6 servings (24 mcgs of VITAMIN K per serving.)

1 1/2	pounds	Shrimp, large
1/4	teaspoon	Red pepper flakes, hot
2	tablespoons	Olive oil, treated (See DIETARY TIP # 10.)
2	tablespoons	Ginger, chopped
1	teaspoon	Garlic, chopped
		Black pepper, ground
1 1/2	cups	Tomatoes, diced
1/4	cup	Scallions, chopped
1/4	cup	Onion

Peel and de-vein the shrimp.

Heat 1 tablespoon of the oil in a frying pan and add the garlic. Cook briefly. Add the tomatoes, hot pepper flakes and 1 tablespoon of the ginger.

Cook, reducing the liquid, for 5 minutes. Set aside and keep warm.

Heat the remaining tablespoon of oil in a nonstick frying pan and add the shrimp and ground pepper. Sauté over high heat for 1 minute on each side.

Add the remaining ginger and the scallions. Blend well, cooking for 1 minute.

Place the shrimp over the tomato mixture and serve.

SEAFOOD STROGANOFF

6 servings (2 mcgs of VITAMIN K per serving.)

1 1/2	pounds	Fillets, salmon
1/4	cup	Butter
3/4	cup	Onion, sliced thin
8	ounces	Mushrooms, sliced
14	ounces	Tomatoes, pear, Italian, crushed
1/2	teaspoon	Salt
1	teaspoon	Worcestershire
1	tablespoon	Lime juice
1	tablespoon	Catsup
1/2	pound	Shrimp, raw, medium
1	cup	Sour cream
2	tablespoons	Flour

Bone, skin, and cut the fish into bite size pieces and set aside.

Melt butter in large frying pan and sauté the onion over medium heat until golden. Add mushrooms. Mix until butter-coated. Add tomatoes, salt, Worcestershire, lime juice, and catsup. Cook, stirring, until liquid is reduced to consistency of thick cream.

Stir in the shrimp. Cover and simmer for 1 minute. Stir in fish and simmer for 2 minutes more.

Blend sour cream with flour until smooth, stir into fish mixture and cook, stirring, until it boils and thickens.

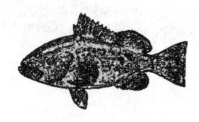

BALSAMIC-GLAZED SALMON FILLETS

6 servings (5 mcgs of VITAMIN K per serving.)

1	teaspoon	Thinly sliced garlic
2	tablespoons	Olive oil, treated (See DIETARY TIP # 10.)
1	teaspoon	Dijon mustard
1	tablespoon	Honey
1/3	cup	Balsamic vinegar
		Salt
		Freshly ground black pepper
6	5 ounce	Salmon fillets, (30 ounces) washed and patted dry with paper towels
2	tablespoons	Fresh basil, julienne cut

In small saucepan, sauté garlic in 1 tablespoon olive oil over medium heat until garlic is tender, about 3 minutes, stirring often. Do not brown. Add the remaining tablespoon of olive oil, mustard, honey, vinegar, 1/4 teaspoon salt and pepper to taste. Stir well to combine. Simmer, uncovered, until slightly thickened, about 3 minutes. Can be made 2 days ahead and refrigerated. Gently reheat before using.

Arrange salmon fillets in single layer on baking pan lined with foil. Brush fillets with warm glaze. Bake on upper oven rack at 475 degrees Fahrenheit until sizzling and glazed, about 10 to 14 minutes, depending on thickness of fillets. Use a fork to pierce the thickest part of fillets to see if it is done. If the fork is hot, the salmon is done! Do not overcook.

Brush with remaining glaze. Season to taste lightly with salt and pepper. Use spatula to transfer to warm serving platter. Garnish fillets with julienne basil

SCALLOPED OYSTERS

8 servings (1 mcg VITAMIN K per serving.)

1/2	cup	Butter
1 1/2	cups	Cracker crumbs
1 1/2	pints	Oysters
		Salt and pepper
		Tabasco
1/2	cup	Oyster liquor
1/2	cup	Cream, heavy
		Buttered bread crumbs

Butter a 1 1/2 to 2 quart baking dish. Cover with a layer of cracker crumbs. Add a layer of half the oysters and another of cracker crumbs. Dot with butter and add seasonings.

Make another layer of oysters and another of cracker crumbs. Dot again with butter and seasonings. Pour the liquids over the top.

Finally sprinkle with buttered bread crumbs.

Bake 25 minutes at 400 degrees Fahrenheit. Serve with beef, turkey, chicken or ham.

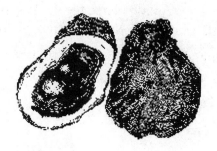

SALMON WITH PISTACHIO-BASIL BUTTER

6 servings (13 mcg of VITAMIN K per serving.)

1/4	cup	Pistachios (about 1 ounce)
6	large	Fresh basil leaves
1	clove	Garlic
1/2	cup	Butter, room temperature
1	teaspoon	Lime juice
6	ounces	1-1/2 inch thick salmon filets
1/2	cup	Dry white wine

Process pistachios, 6 basil leaves and garlic clove in processor until finely chopped. Add 1/2 cup butter and 1 teaspoon lime juice and process until incorporated into mixture. (Toasted almonds could be used instead.) Season to taste with salt and pepper. Transfer butter mixture to small bowl and refrigerate until well chilled (Pistachio butter can be prepared up to 4 days ahead.)

Preheat oven to 400 degrees Fahrenheit.

Butter a 9 by 13 inch baking dish. Place salmon fillets in the dish in a single layer. Pour white wine over salmon. Season salmon with salt and pepper. Bake salmon until almost opaque on top, about 10 minutes.

Place 2 tablespoons pistachio butter on top of each salmon piece. Continue baking until salmon fillets are just opaque in center, about 5 minutes.

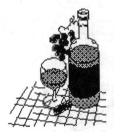

BAKED SALMON WITH FETA VINAIGRETTE

4 servings (5 mcg of VITAMIN K per serving.)

12	ounces	Salmon filets cut into 3 ounce portions
2	tablespoons	Crumbled feta cheese
2 1/2	tablespoons	Lemon juice
1 1/2	tablespoons	Orange juice
1	tablespoon	Water
2	teaspoons	Dijon mustard
2	teaspoons	Oil, olive or Canola, treated (See DIETARY TIP # 10.)
		Additional treated oil for coating the salmon
2	drops	Hot sauce
1/2	cup	Diced red bell pepper

Combine cheese, lemon juice, orange juice, water, Dijon mustard, oil and hot sauce. Stir with a wire whisk.

Preheat the oven to 500 degrees Fahrenheit. Coat each 3 ounce piece with oil. Place on an oiled foil lined pan. Place in the oven at 500 degrees Fahrenheit for 10 to 12 minutes or until a fork, inserted in the thickest part of the filet, feels 'warm to hot,' to the touch.

Top each serving of roasted salmon with 2 tablespoons feta dressing and 2 tablespoons bell pepper.

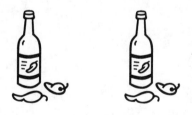

GRILLED FISH IN FOIL

4 servings (9 mcg of VITAMIN K per serving for the sauce. Remember to add the VITAMIN K content for the type of fish you are using.)

This recipe can be used with any of the types of fish we know have a very low amount of VITAMIN K. These include butterfly bream, eel, mackerel, salmon, tuna, and yellowtail (snapper.) However, it will probably taste best with bream, tuna, or yellowtail.

1	pound	Fish fillets
2	tablespoons	Butter
1/4	cup	Lemon juice
1	teaspoon	Fresh dill weed
1	teaspoon	Salt
1/4	teaspoon	Pepper
		Paprika
1	medium	Onion, thinly sliced (about 2/3 cup)

On 4 large buttered squares of heavy-duty aluminum foil, place equal amounts of fish.

In a small saucepan, melt the butter, add the lemon juice, dill weed, salt and pepper and combine thoroughly. Pour equal amounts over fish. Sprinkle with paprika, top with onion slices. Wrap foil securely around fish, leaving space for fish to expand.

Grill 5 to 7 minutes on each side or until fish flakes with fork.

Refrigerate leftovers.

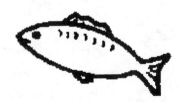

EGGS & CHEESE

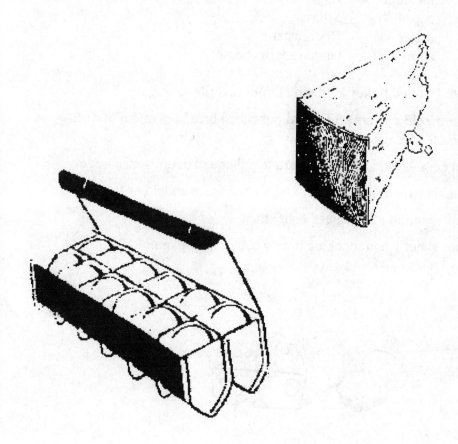

SAUSAGE & EGG CASSEROLE

8 servings (1 mcg of VITAMIN K per serving.)

1	pound	Turkey kielbasa
4	cups	Fresh bread cubes
8	medium	Eggs
2	cups	Milk
1	teaspoon	Dry mustard
1	cup	Grated sharp cheese

Sauté 1 pound turkey kielbasa or your favorite sausage.

Grease 9x13 casserole dish and put cubed bread in bottom of dish. Crumble sausage over bread.

Beat eggs, milk, and dry mustard together and pour over sausage.

Sprinkle with cheese. Cover and refrigerate overnight or freeze.

Bake 1 hour at 350 degrees Fahrenheit.

Takes about 1 hour cooking time whether frozen or not.

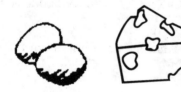

SCOTCH EGGS

12 servings (Less than 2 mcg of VITAMIN K per serving.)

1 1/2	pounds	Sausage or ground beef
1/2	cup	Onion, chopped
2	tablespoons	Steak sauce
1/4	cup	Milk
1/4	cup	To 1/2 cup bread crumbs
1		Egg white, beaten until frothy
6		Hard cooked eggs, shelled (7 eggs if they are small)
1		Egg, slightly beaten
2/3	cup	Bread crumbs or corn flakes crushed
		Other sauce you might want
		Salt and pepper
		Flour

Lightly mix the first six ingredients. Divide into 6 or 7 lumps.

Shape each around an egg, making an oval shape. Roll in flour, then the beaten egg and then the crumbs.

Melt enough oil in a fry pan to make a 2 inch depth. Heat to 325 degrees Fahrenheit. Fry meat rolls, turning once or twice, for five minutes, or until crispy brown. Put in a 325 degree Fahrenheit oven for about 10 to 15 minutes to finish them off.

Then drain on paper towels. Cut in half and serve hot or cold.

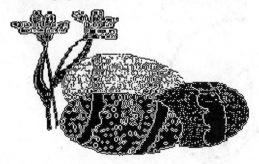

BRUNCH ENCHILADAS

3 servings (2 mcgs of VITAMIN K per serving.) (If salsa is used, add the VITAMIN K content of the salsa.)

3		Tortillas, flour
2	tablespoons	Olive oil, treated (See DIETARY TIP # 10.)
1	cup	Diced ham
2	large	Eggs
1/2	cup	Onion, diced
		Salt
		Black pepper
2	tablespoons	Butter
1/4	cup	White flour
1/2	cup	Colby/jack cheese, shredded
3/4	cup	Milk
		Salsa

Sauté the ham and onion in the olive oil. Add the two eggs and scramble.

In a small pan, heat the butter, and whisk in the flour. Slowly add the milk, while whisking. Heat until thickened and bubbly. Salt and pepper to taste.

Heat the tortillas on a griddle until soft and pliable, but do not allow to harden. Divide the egg mixture into the three tortillas and roll up the tortillas. Pour the white sauce over and top with the cheese. Serve with salsa on the side.

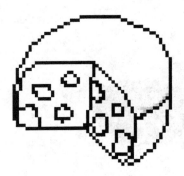

ITALIAN EGGS

4 servings (4 mcg of VITAMIN K per serving.)

1	tablespoon	Olive oil, treated (See DIETARY TIP # 10.)
1	tablespoon	Sweet butter
1	clove	Garlic, smashed
3/4	cup	Onion diced
1/2	pound	Italian turkey sausage
1/2	pound	Beef, extra lean
1	medium	Potato peeled and diced (about 1 cup)
1	cup	Tomato, sliced thin
1/2	teaspoon	Fresh ground pepper
1/3	teaspoon	Salt
8	large	Eggs

Combine olive oil and butter in a skillet and heat. Add onion and garlic and cook until medium brown.

Remove casing from sausage and cut meat into small pieces. Add both sausage and beef to onion. Add diced potato. Cover and cook slowly for 20 minutes.

Add tomato, black pepper and salt and stir. Cook for 15 minutes.

Beat all the eggs together and pour over the top. Cook to taste for 8 to 10 minutes.

Serve with toasted slices of Italian bread.

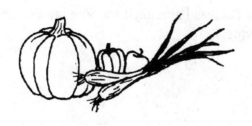

SPICY BREAKFAST SAUSAGE CASSEROLE

12 servings (Less than 2 mcgs of VITAMIN K per serving.)

6	slices	Sourdough bread
2	cups	Cheddar cheese, shredded
1/2	pound	Sausage, hot Italian, cooked and drained
1	cup	Turkey ham or regular ham
1	cup	Mushrooms sliced
1/2	cup	Onion, chopped
10	large	Eggs
2	cups	Milk (to 2 1/2 cups)
2	teaspoons	Salt
1/2	teaspoon	Paprika
1	teaspoon	Fresh oregano
1/2	teaspoon	Black pepper
1/4	teaspoon	Garlic
1/2	teaspoon	Mustard, dry
		Butter

Grease a 9 by 13 pan with butter.

Slice the bread into 1 inch cubes. Put a single, crowded layer of bread into the pan. Dot with butter. Sprinkle shredded cheddar on top of bread. Crumble cooked, drained sausage on top of cheese. Sprinkle with turkey ham, onions, and mushrooms.

Beat eggs and milk together, add salt, paprika, oregano, pepper, garlic and dry mustard. Mix and pour over the cheese in the pan.

Chill at least 12 hours.

Bake uncovered at 325 degrees Fahrenheit for 50 minutes. Let stand for 10 minutes before serving.

SOUPS

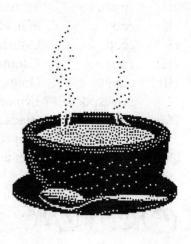

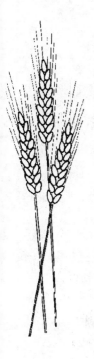

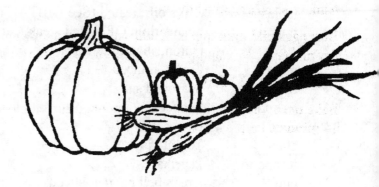

GAZPACHO

6 servings (VITAMIN K content = 13 mcg per cup)

2	cups	Chopped tomatoes
1/2	cup	Finely chopped green pepper
2	cups	Tomato juice
1/2	cup	Fresh basil
1	clove	Garlic, minced
1/2	cup	Chopped cucumber, peeled
1 1/2	cups	Onions, finely chopped
1	tablespoon	Lemon juice
1/4	teaspoon	Black pepper

Combine all ingredients in a mixing bowl and refrigerate. Serve chilled.

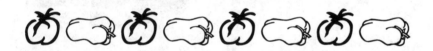

GOULASH SOUP

8 servings (6 mcgs of VITAMIN K per serving.)

2	tablespoons	Olive oil, treated (See DIETARY TIP # 10.)
1	pound	Lean sirloin OR round steak, cut in cubes
1/2	cup	Onion, sliced
2	cloves	Garlic, minced
1	teaspoon	Seasoned salt
1/4	teaspoon	Pepper
3 3/4	cups	Beef broth
3	cups	Tomato juice
1	teaspoon	Paprika
1/2	cup	Green bell pepper, sliced
8	ounces	Extra wide egg noodles, uncooked

In a large kettle or Dutch oven, heat the oil. Add meat, onion, garlic, salt, and pepper.

Cook and stir until meat is browned. Add next three ingredients, simmer covered 20 to 30 minutes until meat is tender.

Bring broth to boil. Stir in bell peppers and egg noodles. Cook on low boil 10 minutes until noodles are tender.

Refrigerate leftovers.

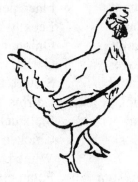

SHERRIED CHICKEN SOUP
6 servings (2 mcg of VITAMIN K per serving.)

1	large	Chicken breast
1/2	cup	Green pepper, cut in thin strips
1/2	cup	Mushrooms, sliced
1/4	cup	Flour
1/2	cup	Sherry
1	cup	Chicken broth
2 1/2	cups	Cream (half and half)

Pressure cook chicken for 12 minutes with 1 cup water, salt and pepper to taste with a piece of celery and onion for flavor. Or you can poach on stove top until chicken is done. Approximately 20 minutes.

Reserve broth and cut chicken into bite size pieces.

Sauté green pepper and mushrooms lightly in a bit of the butter.

Make a white sauce with the rest of the butter (melted), flour and half and half.

Thin with broth and add mushrooms, green pepper and chicken. Heat without boiling, add sherry and serve.

This is equally good chilled.

OLD-FASHIONED CHICKEN SOUP

6 servings (21 mcgs of VITAMIN K per serving.)

2 1/2	pounds	Chicken cut into serving pieces, (sprinkle with black pepper, paprika and onion powder)
1	cup	Leek, white and 1 1/2 inch green part, thinly sliced
1	Large	Onion, chopped (about 1 cup)
4	cloves	Garlic, minced
1	pound	Stewed tomatoes, chopped, undrained
1 1/2	cups	Carrots, peeled, thinly sliced
1/2	cup	Stalk celery, thinly sliced
6	cups	Chicken broth
		White pepper to taste
2	medium	Potatoes, peeled, cubed, cooked
2	tablespoons	Chives, chopped

In a 9x13-inch baking pan, bake chicken at 350-degrees Fahrenheit for 40 minutes. (This seals in the juices and takes the place of browning the chicken in oil, reducing the amount of oil needed. It will also de-fat the chicken).

Meanwhile, in a Dutch oven casserole, cook together the next 8 ingredients for 40 minutes. Add the chicken to the casserole, discarding the skin, bones and fat in the pan. Continue cooking for 15 minutes, or until chicken is tender. Add the potatoes and heat through. Sprinkle with chives.

CHICKEN AND RICE SOUP

4 servings (Less than 1 mcg of VITAMIN K per serving.)

2	cups	Chicken broth
3	cups	Water
1	tablespoon	Lemon juice
1	clove	Garlic
1/2	cup	Long-grain white rice
1	pound	Chicken breast, boneless, skinless
		Salt and pepper

Combine chicken broth, water and lemon juice in a saucepan. Peel the garlic and drop it in. Cover the pan and bring to a boil over high heat. Add the rice, cover, and simmer over medium heat until rice is soft, about 15 minutes.

Meanwhile cut the chicken into thin shreds. When rice is tender, add the chicken, cover and continue to simmer until the chicken is cooked through, about 5 minutes. Fish out the garlic clove and season the soup to taste with salt and pepper.

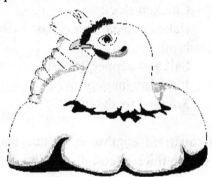

CHICKEN SOUP
8 servings (5 mcgs of VITAMIN K per serving.)

3	pounds	Chicken, cut up
1	pound	Potatoes, washed
1	cup	Carrots, diced
1	cup	Celery, chopped with leaves
1	cup	Onion, chopped
1	tablespoon	Salt
6	cups	Water
6		Peppercorns
1		Bay leaf

Layer chicken and potatoes, carrots, celery and onion in crock pot. Sprinkle salt between layers and add water.

Tie peppercorns and bay leaf in a piece of cheesecloth. Push under liquid.

Cook on low 8 hours, or high 4 hours, until chicken is tender.

BAKED POTATO CHICKEN SOUP

6 servings (Less than 1 mcg of VITAMIN K per serving without the chives. 6 mcgs of VITAMIN K per serving with the chives.)

2	large	Baking potatoes, cooked and cooled (about 2 pounds)
1/2	cup	Ham, diced (Prosciutto would be good here.)
2	tablespoons	Olive oil, treated (See DIETARY TIP # 10.)
1/2	cup	Onion, chopped
4	cups	Chicken stock
1 1/2	cups	Baked cooked chicken or 2 cans chunk chicken in-broth
		Salt and pepper, to taste
2	tablespoons	Plain lowfat yogurt
1	tablespoon	Snipped fresh chives

Cut the potatoes into quarters lengthwise, do not remove the skins. Cut each quarter into 1/4-inch thick slices, discarding the end slices, and set the potatoes aside.

Sauté the ham in the oil in a deep saucepan over medium heat until crisp and slightly browned. Remove the ham with a slotted spoon and drain on paper towels. Pour off all but 1 tablespoon of the oil.

Add the onion to the saucepan and sauté until translucent. Add the stock and bring to boiling.

Add the potatoes and the chicken. Simmer the soup for 5 minutes, stirring once or twice, to heat the chicken and the potatoes. Season the soup with salt and pepper.

Garnish the soup with the ham, yogurt and chives.

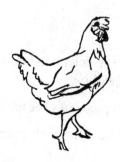

ITALIAN VEGETABLE SOUP WITH PROSCIUTTO

10 servings (76 mcgs of VITAMIN K per serving.)

2	tablespoons	Olive oil, treated (See DIETARY TIP # 10.)
3/4	cup	Onion, diced
1	large	Garlic clove, minced
6	cups	Water
28	ounces	Canned tomatoes, chopped (liquid reserved)
1	cup	Carrots, peeled and sliced
1	cup	Celery, sliced
2	cups	Sliced cabbage
4	ounces	Prosciutto, diced very fine
1/2	cup	Dry red wine
		Salt and pepper
16	ounces	Kidney beans, canned, drained
1	cup	Zucchini, peeled and sliced
1/2	cup	Pennette or other tube shaped pasta
		Freshly grated Parmesan cheese

Heat oil in heavy large saucepan over high heat.

Add onion and garlic and sauté until garlic is brown, about 45 seconds.

Add next 8 ingredients. Season with salt and pepper. Bring mixture to boil. Reduce heat and simmer, stirring occasionally for 1 hour.

Mix beans, zucchini and pasta into soup. Simmer until pasta and zucchini are tender, about 15 minutes.

Serve hot, passing cheese separately.

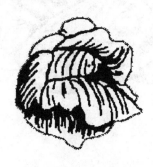

TOMATO-BEEF SOUP

8 servings (8 mcgs of VITAMIN K per serving.)

1	pound	Ground beef
1	cup	Chopped onion
1/2	cup	Chopped celery
1	tablespoon	Butter
3	cups	Tomatoes
2		Beef bouillon cubes
1/3	cup	Long grain uncooked rice
1	teaspoon	Salt
1/2	teaspoon	Chili powder
1		Bay leaf
3 1/2	cups	Water

Sauté beef, onion and celery in melted butter until meat is browned. Stir in remaining ingredients.

Bring to a boil. Reduce heat, cover and simmer for 20 minutes. Remove bay leaf.

Makes 2 quarts of hearty soup.

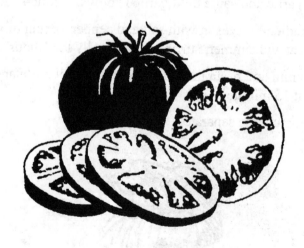

TEX-MEX BEEF SOUP

4 servings (18 mcgs of VITAMIN K per serving.)

1/2	pound	Beef round steak, boneless, cut into 1/2 inch cubes
1	cup	Onion, chopped
1	clove	Garlic, minced
2	cups	Water
16	ounces	Tomatoes, cut up
1	cup	Carrot, chopped
8	ounces	Kidney beans, canned, drained
1/2	cup	Green pepper, chopped
1/2	cup	Tomato puree
1	tablespoon	Chili powder
2	teaspoons	Beef bouillon granules
1/4	teaspoon	Pepper
		Canola oil for pan, treated (See DIETARY TIP # 10.)

Oil a large saucepan with Canola oil. Preheat over medium-high heat.

Add beef, onion, and garlic. Cook and stir about 3 minutes or until meat is brown.

Stir in water, undrained tomatoes, carrot, beans, green pepper, tomato paste, chili powder, bouillon granules, and pepper. Cover and simmer about 30 minutes or until meat is tender. Serve.

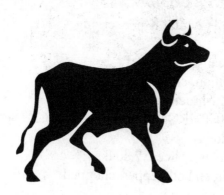

VEGETABLE-BEEF SOUP

16 cup servings (31 mcgs of VITAMIN K per serving.)

2		Beef soup bones
8	cups	Water
1 1/2	pounds	Stew beef, cut into 1 inch cubes
1 1/2	teaspoon	Salt
1	teaspoon	Pepper
4	medium	Potatoes, cubed
1	cup	Carrots, cubed
1	cup	Onions, coarsely chopped
16	ounces	Tomato sauce
1	cup	Cabbage, coarsely chopped
17	ounces	Canned corn, drained
2	cups	Green peas, drained

Combine soup bones and water in a large Dutch oven and bring to a boil. Cover, reduce heat, and simmer 1 hour.

Add beef cubes, salt, and pepper, cover and simmer 1 hour.

Add potatoes, carrots, onions, tomato sauce, hot pepper, and cabbage, cover and simmer 40 minutes.

Add corn and peas, simmer, uncovered, 30 minutes.

CREAMY BEEF-NOODLE COMBO

5 servings (11 mcgs of VITAMIN K per serving.)

1	pound	Lean ground beef
1/2	cup	Onion, chopped, 1 medium
4	ounces	Mushrooms, stems and pieces
1 1/4	cups	MUSHROOM CREAM SAUCE (See Recipe Index)
1	cup	Celery, sliced, 2 stalks
1/2	cup	Green bell pepper, chopped
1/4	cup	Pimento, sliced
1	cup	Milk
1	tablespoon	Worcestershire sauce

| 1 | teaspoon | Salt |
| 4 | ounces | Noodles, uncooked, about 2 cups |

Cook and stir the meat and onion in a large skillet until the meat is brown. Drain off the excess fat.

Stir in the UNDRAINED mushroom pieces and the remaining ingredients. Heat to boiling then reduce the heat and simmer, covered, stirring occasionally, until the noodles are tender, about 25 minutes. A small amount of water can be added if necessary. Serve hot.

RED FISH CHOWDER

6 servings (7 mcgs of VITAMIN K per serving.)

2	tablespoons	Butter,
1	clove	Garlic, minced
1	medium	Onion, diced (about 1/2 cup)
1/2	cup	Green pepper, diced
1/2	cup	Celery rib, diced
1	cup	Crushed tomatoes
1	cup	Dry red wine
1	pound	Haddock
3	cups	Potatoes, diced
6	cups	Water
		Salt, pepper
		Tabasco and Worcestershire

Melt butter in stock pot and sauté garlic, onion, green pepper and celery until tender, stirring often.

Add water, fish, tomatoes, wine and potatoes. Season to taste and bring to a boil and cook until the potatoes and fish are tender.

SOPA DE PESCADO (FISH)

8 servings (5 mcgs of VITAMIN K per serving.)

2	quarts	Fish stock*
1	cup	Cooked shrimp, pieces
2	tablespoons	Lemon juice
1/2	pound	Vermicelli noodles, uncooked
1		Hard boiled egg, cubed
		GREEN CHILE SAUCE (See Recipe Index)
		Croutons or other garnish

*Can be liquid from boiled fish, seasoned with a few drops of olive oil, onion, bay leaf and salt.

Heat broth, add shellfish, lemon juice and vermicelli noodles, simmer until heated through and pasta is al dente. Serve with a small dollop of GREEN CHILE SAUCE (See Recipe Index) in each dish. To be stirred in by the diner.

Garnish with the egg and croutons

GREEN CHILE SAUCE

8 servings (3 mcgs of VITAMIN K per serving.)

2	tablespoons	Oil, olive or Canola treated (SEE DIETARY TIP # 10.)
1	clove	Garlic
1/2	cup	Minced onion
1	tablespoon	Flour
1	cup	Water
1	cup	Diced green chili
		Salt to taste

In oil in a heavy saucepan, sauté garlic and onion. Blend in flour with wooden spoon. Add water and green chili. Bring to a boil and simmer, stirring frequently, for 5 minutes.

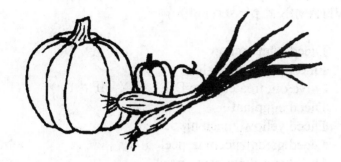

QUICK FISH CHOWDER

4 servings (8 mcgs of VITAMIN K per serving.)

3	tablespoons	Olive oil, treated (See DIETARY TIP # 10.)
1/2	cup	Onion, chopped
2	stalks	Celery, sliced, about 3/4 cup
1	teaspoon	Chili powder
1	pound	Canned stewed tomatoes and juice
1	cup	Water or fish stock
1	teaspoon	Salt
1	teaspoon	Sugar
1	teaspoon	Worcestershire sauce
1	pound	Haddock, snapper or bream, cut into chunks
		Garlic croutons for garnish

Heat oil in saucepan. Pitch in onion, celery, and chili powder. Sauté over medium heat for 10 minutes.

Stir in tomatoes, water, salt, sugar, and Worcestershire sauce. Bring to a rolling boil and add fish. Reduce heat and simmer, covered, for about 15 minutes. Sprinkle with garlic croutons.

TOMATO BISQUE

6 cups (17 mcgs of VITAMIN K per serving.)

1	cup	Diced white onion
1	teaspoon	Finely chopped garlic
3	tablespoons	Olive oil, treated (See DIETARY TIP # 10.)
1	cup	Diced eggplant
1	cup	Diced yellow zucchini, peeled
1	cup	Diced green zucchini, peeled
1	cup	Diced sweet peppers, green
1/4	cup	Tomato puree
1 1/3	cups	Tomato juice
1 1/3	cups	Chicken stock
6	leaves	Chopped fresh basil leaves
		Salt and pepper

Cook onion and garlic in hot oil for 2 minutes. Add eggplant, zucchini and peppers. Cook 5 minutes.

Add tomato paste and cook 5 minutes on low heat. Stir in tomato juice and stock. Simmer until vegetables are just tender, about 8 to 10 minutes.

Stir in basil, season with salt and pepper.

CARROT VICHYSSOISE

6 servings (19 mcgs of VITAMIN K per serving.)

2	cups	Chopped, peeled potatoes
1 1/2	cups	Sliced carrots
3	cups	Leeks, white part and green part, sliced
5	cups	Chicken broth
1	teaspoon	Salt
1	dash	White pepper
1	cup	Half and half
		Sour cream

Combine potatoes, carrots, leeks and broth in large saucepan. Bring to boil, then simmer, uncovered, 25 minutes or until vegetables are tender.

Puree vegetables and liquid, half at a time, in blender. Empty into mixing bowl. Stir in salt, white pepper and half and half. Chill well. Serve in cups or mugs, garnished with dollop of sour cream.

VEGETABLE SOUP

8 servings (24 mcgs of VITAMIN K per serving.)

8	cups	Low-fat chicken broth
1	cup	Carrots, diced
1	cup	Celery, chopped
1	cup	Onion, sliced
3	cloves	Garlic, minced
1	tablespoon	Fresh basil, chopped
2	cups	Green beans, (fresh or frozen)
2	cups	Yellow summer squash, peeled and diced
2	small	Zucchini, peeled and diced
1	cup	White beans, cooked
1	cup	Corn, cut
	dash	Ground pepper, or to taste

Please note: This may be made ahead and frozen.

Combine broth, carrots, celery, onion, garlic, and basil in large pot. Bring to boil and simmer 30 minutes. Add green beans, yellow squash, zucchini and beans. Simmer 30 minutes. Add corn and cook 20 minutes longer. Season to taste. Makes 6 to 8 servings.

Variations: Add 1 cup pasta along with the corn, or add 1 cup barley in the beginning.

BEEF AND LENTIL STEW

6 servings (14 mcgs of VITAMIN K per serving.)

1	pound	Beef, lean, ground
1/2	cup	Onion, chopped, 1 medium
1	clove	Garlic, minced
4	ounces	Mushroom stems and pieces
16	ounces	Stewed tomatoes
1/2	cup	Celery, sliced
1/2	cup	Carrot, sliced
1	cup	Lentils, uncooked
3	cups	Water
1/4	cup	Red Wine, Optional
1		Bay leaf
1	teaspoon	Salt
1	teaspoon	Beef bouillon, instant
1/4	teaspoon	Pepper

Cook and stir the meat, onion and garlic in a Dutch oven until the meat is brown. Drain off the excess fat.

Stir in the undrained mushrooms, and the remaining ingredients. Heat to boiling, then reduce the heat, cover, and simmer, stirring occasionally, until the lentils are tender, about 40 minutes.

Remove the bay leaf and serve.

PUREE OF CARROT SOUP

6 servings (4 mcgs of VITAMIN K per serving.)

1	pound	Carrots, peeled and thinly sliced
1	cup	Onions, chopped
1	tablespoon	Oil, olive or Canola, treated (See DIETARY TIP # 10.)
2	tablespoons	Butter
4	cups	Chicken broth
		Salt and pepper to taste

Heat a large saucepan. Add butter and oil and sauté onions until golden. Add carrots and chicken broth and simmer gently until carrots are tender. Puree in a blender, return to pan and thin (or not) with additional chicken broth. You could add some heavy cream or evaporated skim milk if you wanted a creamed soup. Bring to a boil, garnish with a sprig of dill and serve.

CARROT HORSERADISH SOUP
4 servings (6 mcgs of VITAMIN K per serving.)

2	tablespoons	Oil, olive or Canola, treated (See DIETARY TIP # 10.)
1	small	Onion, minced
1/2	cup	Celery, minced
1	clove	Garlic, minced
1	cup	Carrots, finely diced
20	ounces	Beef consommé or broth
6	ounces	Water
1	tablespoon	Prepared horseradish
2	teaspoons	Butter
2	teaspoons	Flour
		Pepper to taste

In saucepan, heat oil and add onions, celery, and garlic. Lightly sauté until onion is transparent, about 5 minutes.

Add carrots, consommé and water. Cover tightly, bring to a boil, reduce heat and simmer until carrots are tender, about 15 minutes.

Add horseradish. Combine butter and flour into a paste, then drop (in small bits) into gently simmering soup. Cook, stirring, until mixture is absorbed and very lightly thickened. Taste for seasoning and add dash of pepper if desired. Serve hot.

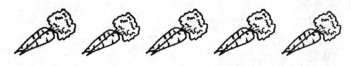

CARROT POTATO CHOWDER
6 servings (2 mcgs of VITAMIN K per serving.)

3/4	cup	White onion, minced
1/4	cup	Butter
2	cups	Diced raw potatoes
3	cups	Boiling water
1	teaspoon	Salt
1/4	teaspoon	Paprika
1	tablespoon	Flour
2	cups	Milk, scalded
3/4	cup	Carrots, diced and cooked

Sauté onion in 2 tablespoons of butter in large saucepan until lightly browned.

Add potatoes, boiling water, salt and paprika. Boil about 15 minutes or until potatoes are soft.

Blend flour with remaining butter and gradually add milk, stirring constantly, until smooth and thickened.

Add to potato mixture. Add carrots. Cook 5 minutes, stirring until smooth.

SAUSAGE CHOWDER
6 servings (3 mcgs of VITAMIN K per serving.)

1	pound	Smoked sausage, cut in chunks
1	cup	Onion, chopped
3	large	Potatoes, peeled and diced
2	teaspoons	Salt
1	teaspoon	Fresh basil, chopped
1/8	teaspoon	Pepper
2	cups	Water
1	can	Cream style corn
1	can	Whole kernel corn
18	ounces	Evaporated milk

Brown Sausage. Add onion and sauté without browning. Add potatoes, seasonings and water.

Cover, simmer 15 minutes. Stir in corn and milk. Heat to boiling point. Do not let boil!

Serve hot.

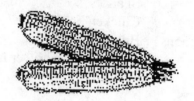

CORN CHOWDER

11 servings (2 mcgs of VITAMIN K per serving.)

3	slices	Bacon, diced
4	cups	Chicken broth
1	pound	Chicken, cut in 1/2 inch cubes
3/4	cup	Onion, minced
3/4	cup	Celery, finely chopped
4	cups	Corn, whole kernel (divided)
2	cups	Potatoes, diced
1/2	teaspoon	Salt
1	cup	Cream, heavy
1/8	teaspoon	Pepper, white

In Dutch oven, over medium heat, cook bacon until crisp. Remove with slotted spoon and pour off all but 2 tablespoons of the drippings. Add chicken, onion, celery and cook 10-15 minutes or until tender.

In blender, combine 1 cup chicken broth and 2 cups of corn. Blend on high until smooth. Stir into Dutch oven along with remaining corn, potatoes and chicken broth. Add salt and bring to boil. Reduce heat and simmer partially covered 20 minutes or until potatoes are tender.

Stir in cream and pepper and simmer 2-3 minutes more. Stir in bacon and serve.

MUSHROOM SOUP

6 servings (Less than 1 mcg of VITAMIN K per serving.)

1	pound	Mushrooms
2		Shallots
4	cups	Chicken broth
4	tablespoons	Butter
6	slices	French bread, dry, crusts removed
1/2	cup	Cream

Wash and dry the mushrooms. Chop about 3/4 pound and slice the rest. Chop the shallots very finely.

In a soup kettle, melt 3 tablespoons of the butter and sauté the shallots until tender. Add the chopped mushrooms and continue cooking 5 minutes, stirring occasionally.

Pour in the chicken broth, season with salt and pepper and cook slowly for 30 minutes, uncovered.

Meanwhile, with the remaining 1 tablespoon of butter, sauté the sliced mushrooms on high heat with a teaspoon of lemon juice and a pinch of salt.

Make bread crumbs with the dry bread. Add the bread crumbs to the soup and continue cooking 8 more minutes.

When ready to serve, add the cream and the reserved sliced mushrooms to the hot soup.

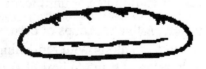

BEAN SOUP

8 servings (5 mcgs of VITAMIN K per serving.)

1	pounds	Navy beans,
1	pound	Pinto beans
1	pound	Green split peas
1	pound	Black eyed peas
1	pound	Lentils
1	pound	Large limas
1	pound	Red kidney beans
1	pound	Barley
6 3/4	cups	Chicken stock
2	cups	Garlic
1/4	teaspoon	Pepper
		Salt to taste
3	cups	Ham, diced and cooked
1	large	Onion, chopped (about 1 cup)
16	ounces	Tomatoes, undrained and chopped
3	tablespoons	Lime juice

This is a recipe for Bean Soup. (It is meant to be used for gifts.)

One pound each of the seven varieties of beans and the barley are to be mixed together and then divided into 10 (1 1/2 cup) portions. Each portion is packed for gift giving. (Mason jar, cloth sack, etc.)

Include the following directions with each gift portion of beans.

Sort and wash the beans, place in Dutch oven. Cover with water 2 inches above level of beans and soak overnight. Drain off water, leave the beans in the Dutch oven, add broth and pepper. Cover and bring to a boil. Reduce heat and simmer 1 1/2 hours or until beans are tender. Add remaining ingredients and simmer, uncovered, 30 minutes, stirring occasionally.

Serve hot. Yield 2 1/2 quarts.

WHITE GAZPACHO

6 servings (4 mcgs of VITAMIN K per serving.)

4	teaspoon	Instant chicken bouillon OR
4	cubes	Chicken bouillon
2	cups	Boiling water
3	medium	Cucumbers, peeled
16	ounces	Sour cream
2	tablespoons	Lemon juice
1/4	teaspoon	Garlic powder
1/4	teaspoon	Pepper

Pare and seed the cucumbers. Cut into cubes so that you have about 3 cups of cubes.

In small saucepan, dissolve bouillon in water. Cool completely. In blender or food processor, blend peeled cucumber with 1/2 cup bouillon liquid until smooth.

In medium bowl, combine cucumber mixture, remaining bouillon liquid, sour cream, lemon juice, garlic powder and pepper, mix well. Chill thoroughly.

Garnish as desired. Serve with condiments. Refrigerate leftovers.

SUGGESTED CONDIMENTS:

Chopped fresh tomato, chopped red onions, chopped green peppers, toasted slivered almonds or toasted croutons. Use 1/4 cup garnish per serving.

STRAW MUSHROOM SOUP

2 servings (80 mcgs of VITAMIN K per serving.)

14	ounces	Chicken broth
1/4	cup	Dry sherry
1/8	teaspoon	White pepper
1/3	cup	Straw mushrooms, canned
1	teaspoon	Sesame oil
1/3	cup	Scallions, sliced

In small saucepan, combine chicken broth, sherry and white pepper. Bring to a boil, reduce heat and add mushrooms and sesame oil. Heat for a minute.

Just before serving, sprinkle with scallions.

POTATO SOUP

4 servings (10 mcgs of VITAMIN K per serving.)

2	medium	Potatoes
1	medium	Onion
1 1/2	cups	Celery stalks and leaves
2	tablespoons	Olive or Canola oil, treated (See DIETARY TIP # 10.)
		Boiling water
1	small	Bay leaf
1/2	teaspoon	Salt
2	tablespoons	Butter
2	cups	Milk, up to 3 cups may be used

Peel and thinly slice potatoes, onion and celery.

Sauté for 3 to 5 minutes in hot vegetable oil.

In a large pot, add all of the vegetables and cover with just enough boiling water to cover. Place bay leaf and salt in pot and boil vegetables until tender.

Drain vegetables and reserve liquid. Mash vegetables into vegetable stock and add butter.

Thin soup with milk as desired, heat until warm. (DO NOT boil.) Ladle into soup bowls.

SWEET SQUASH BISQUE

6 servings (6 mcg of VITAMIN K per serving.)

1	teaspoon	Olive oil, treated (See DIETARY TIP # 10.)
1	cup	Celery, minced
1	cup	Onion, minced
2 1/4	cups	Winter squash, peeled, seeded and diced
1	large	Potato, peeled and diced
1	large	Pear, peeled, cored, diced
3	can	Vegetable broth
1	cup	Water
1/4	teaspoon	Ground cumin
1/4	teaspoon	Fresh grated nutmeg
1/4	cup	Half-and-half, optional
		Salt and fresh ground pepper

Heat oil in 3-quart pot over medium to high heat. When hot, add celery and onion. Cook until hot and fragrant, about 3 minutes. Add squash, potato, pear, broth, water, cumin and nutmeg. Simmer, covered, until squash and potato are soft, about 25 minutes.

Strain vegetables from cooking liquid, reserving both. Puree solids in food processor or in blender until completely smooth, about 2 minutes. Add 1/2 cup reserved liquid to food processor to make mixture smoother. Return pureed mixture and reserved liquid to pot. Add half- and-half. Heat through. Season to taste with salt and pepper. Can be made 3 days ahead and refrigerated, or frozen as long as 4 months. Gently reheat. Serve hot.

FRUIT SOUP

4 servings (10 mcgs of VITAMIN K per serving.)

1 1/3	cups	Apricot nectar
2	teaspoons	Cornstarch
2	tablespoons	Brandy
2	tablespoons	Honey
1/8	teaspoon	Ground allspice
1 1/2	cups	Peaches, pineapples, apricots and plums

In a nonmetal bowl, stir together apricot nectar and cornstarch. Stir in brandy, honey, and allspice.

Micro-cook, uncovered, on 100% power for 2 to 3 minutes or until the mixture is thickened and bubbly, stirring every 30 seconds. Stir in fruit. Micro-cook, uncovered, on 100% power for 45 seconds to 1 minute or until heated through.

Chill thoroughly, if desired. Serve hot or cold.

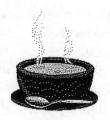

TOMATO SOUP

8 servings (10 mcgs of VITAMIN K per serving.)

1/2	cup	Onion, chopped
1	tablespoon	Olive oil, treated (See DIETARY TIP # 10.)
3	cloves	Garlic, chopped
1	Stick	Butter
1/2	cup	Flour
28	ounces	Canned, crushed tomatoes
1	cup	Fresh tomato, finely chopped
1	quart	Chicken stock, heated
1	pint	Half-and-half or milk
		Salt and pepper to taste
		Croutons for garnish

Sauté onions in olive oil until translucent. Add garlic and butter. When butter is melted, add flour and stir until smooth. Add crushed tomatoes with juice, fresh tomatoes and heated stock, bring to a boil, reduce heat and simmer 5 minutes.

Scald cream or milk (in heavy saucepan, heat cream or milk gently, just until bubbles are seen at the edge of the pan, do not allow to boil). Stir scalded milk into soup and add salt and pepper to taste.

FRENCH ONION SOUP
6 servings (Less than 1 mcg of VITAMIN K per serving.)

4	medium	Onions, thinly sliced
4	tablespoons	Butter
1	tablespoon	Olive oil, treated (See DIETARY TIP # 10.)
1 1/2	teaspoon	Salt
1	tablespoon	Granulated sugar
3	tablespoons	All-purpose flour
2	cans	(15 1/2 ounce each) beef broth
1	tablespoon	Beef bouillon crystals
1	cup	Dry white wine
1/2	cup	Brandy
1/2	teaspoon	Salt
1/2	teaspoon	Freshly ground pepper
4	cups	Water

To caramelize onions, place onions, butter, and oil in large saucepan over medium heat. Cover and cook, stirring occasionally, 20 minutes. Stir in 1 1/2 teaspoon salt, sugar, and flour. Cook uncovered 40 minutes, stirring frequently. Stir in beef broth, bouillon, wine, brandy, salt and pepper, and water. Bring to a boil, reduce heat, and simmer 40 minutes.

Ladle into oven-proof serving bowls, top with a slice of toasted French bread and grated Swiss cheese (Gruyere is best). Place under broiler just until cheese is melted and bubbly.

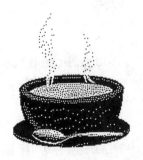

HUNGARIAN STYLE SOUP

6 servings (6 mcgs of VITAMIN K per serving.)

1/4	pound	Bacon, in 1 inch pieces
4	medium	Onions, chopped
1	pound	Beef, lean, cut into 1/2 inch cubes
6	cups	Beef broth
16	ounces	Tomatoes, canned
1/4	cup	Red wine
1	tablespoon	Tomato paste
1	clove	Garlic minced
2	teaspoons	Paprika
1/2	teaspoon	Caraway seeds
1/4	teaspoon	Marjoram, fresh chopped
1	teaspoon	Salt
1/4	teaspoon	Pepper
1/2	teaspoon	Sugar
1	pound	Potatoes, diced
3/4	pound	Kielbasa, knockwurst, etc., sliced

Cook bacon until transparent. Add onion and cook until golden.

Add the beef and cook until it's lost its red color.

Add the remaining ingredients except for the potatoes and sausage.

Bring to a boil. Simmer covered for 30 minutes.

Add the potatoes and sliced sausage. Cook for about 30 minutes until potatoes are tender. Skim off fat. Serve hot.

HEARTY CHICKEN AND RICE SOUP
8 servings (6 mcgs of VITAMIN K per serving.)

10	cups	Chicken broth
1	medium	Onion
1	cup	Sliced celery
1	cup	Sliced carrots
1/4	teaspoon	Cracked black pepper
1/2	teaspoon	Fresh thyme leaves
1		Bay leaf
1 1/2	cups	Cubed chicken - (3/4 pound)
2	cups	Cooked rice
2	tablespoons	Lime juice
		Lime slices, for garnish

Combine broth, onion, celery, carrots, pepper, thyme, and bay leaf in Dutch oven. Bring to a boil, stir once or twice. Reduce heat and simmer, uncovered, 10 to 15 minutes.

Add the chicken and simmer, uncovered, 5 to 10 minutes or until chicken is cooked. Remove and discard bay leaf.

Stir in rice and lime juice just before serving.

Garnish with lime slices.

MINESTRONE SOUP
10 to 20 servings (VITAMIN K content = 68 mcg per cup)

2	cups	Uncooked. plain pasta
10	cups	Water
6	ounces	Tomato paste
1	clove	Minced garlic
1/4	cup	Olive oil, treated (See DIETARY TIP # 10.)
1 1/2	cups	Chopped onions
1 1/2	cups	Chopped celery
1	teaspoon	Fresh chopped parsley
1	cup	Chopped carrots
4 1/2	cups	Shredded cabbage

2	cups	Chopped tomatoes
1	cup	Red kidney beans
1 1/2	cups	Green peas
1 1/2	cups	Fresh green beans

Sauté garlic and onions in olive oil. Add all remaining ingredients except pasta and mix. Bring to boil and cover.

Cook on low heat for 45 minutes to an hour until vegetables are at desired tenderness. Add uncooked pasta and cook until pasta is al dente.

WINTER SQUASH, APPLE AND WALNUT SOUP
6 servings (5 mcgs of VITAMIN K per serving.)

24	ounces	Butternut squash, peeled, cooked and pureed
2	tablespoons	Unsalted butter
1	cup	Unsweetened applesauce
1	cup	Light cream
1 1/2	cups	Chicken stock
1/4	cup	Ground toasted walnuts
1/2	teaspoon	Ground mace
		Salt
		White pepper
1/2	cup	Toasted walnut pieces for garnish

Combine all the ingredients (except the walnuts) in a large saucepan and stir to blend well. Cook the soup over medium heat until warmed through, about 6 to 8 minutes.

Ladle the soup into bowls and add a few chopped walnut pieces in the center.

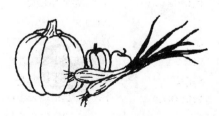

GOLDEN MUSTARD SQUASH SOUP

6 servings (8 mcgs of VITAMIN K per serving. 11 mcgs of VITAMIN K per serving with chives.)

1/4	cup	Butter
1	cup	Onion, chopped
1/2	cup	Carrot, peeled and chopped
1/3	cup	Celery stalk, chopped
3	cups	Chicken broth
2	cups	Beef broth
1 1/2	pounds	Yellow summer squash, peeled and diced
1	medium	Potato, peeled and diced
3/4	cup	Whipping cream
1 1/2	tablespoons	Dijon mustard
1/2	teaspoon	Nutmeg, fresh grated
		Salt and white pepper
1/3	cup	Freshly grated carrot and
2	teaspoons	Snipped fresh chives for garnish

Melt butter in heavy large saucepan over low heat. Add onion, carrot and celery. Cover and cook until onion is translucent, about 10 minutes, stir occasionally.

Add chicken and beef broth, squash and potato. Increase heat to high and bring to simmer. Let simmer until vegetable mixture is very tender, about 30 minutes.

Transfer mixture to processor or blender in batches and puree until smooth. Pour into bowl. (For finer texture, strain soup.) Stir in cream, mustard and nutmeg. Salt and pepper to taste. Cover and refrigerate. Taste and adjust seasoning. Garnish with carrot and chives just before serving.

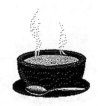

RICE PASTA & POTATOES

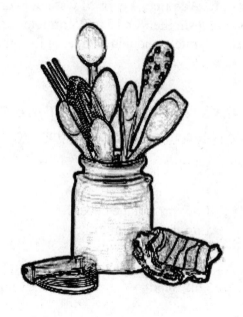

TASTY WHITE RICE WITH CORN

8 servings (This recipe essentially contains no vitamin K. The corn is optional.)

4	cups	Water
2	cups	White rice
1	tablespoon	Canola or olive oil, treated (See DIETARY TIP # 10.)
2	cloves	Minced garlic
1/2	teaspoons	Salt
1/2	cup	Corn, frozen or fresh

Sauté onion and garlic. Add rice, 4 cups of water and bring to a boil. Reduce heat. Cover and simmer for 15 to 25 minutes or until rice is cooked. Cook corn separately and add to rice, onion and garlic mixture.

BAKED POTATOES STUFFED WITH COTTAGE CHEESE

4 servings (VITAMIN K content = less than 1 mcg per 1/2 potato, with or without skin.)

4		Baking potatoes
3/4	cup	Low-fat cottage cheese
1/4	cup	Low-fat or skim milk
1	tablespoon	Butter
2	teaspoons	Grated parmesan cheese
1	teaspoon	Dill weed

Bake potatoes in oven for 1 hour at 400 degrees Fahrenheit or until tender. Remove potatoes from oven and cut in half. Remove potato flesh and put in bowl. Add all other ingredients to make mixture. Place mixture back into potato skins. Bake for 15 minutes until top is golden brown.

RAW POTATO LOAF

4 servings (14 mcgs of vitamin K per serving.)

4	cups	Grated raw potatoes
1	cup	Onion grated with potatoes
1/2	cup	Flour
4	tablespoons	Canned evaporated milk
1		Egg (beaten into the canned milk)
1 1/2	teaspoon	Baking powder
1	teaspoon	Salt
1/4	teaspoon	Pepper

Mix all ingredients together. Place in loaf pan. Put dabs of butter on top of potatoes before putting in oven. Bake 60 minutes in 350 degrees Fahrenheit oven. You can also use the mixture for potato pancakes instead of the loaf.

MACARONI AND CHEESE

4 servings (VITAMIN K content = 2 mcg per cup)

1/2	cup	Evaporated skim milk
2	cups	Macaroni
1	large	Egg, beaten
1/4	teaspoon	Black pepper
1 1/4	cups	Shredded sharp white cheddar cheese

Cook macaroni, drain, and set aside.

Grease baking pan with 1/4 teaspoon Canola or olive oil. Combine all ingredients, including macaroni, in mixing bowl. After thoroughly mixed, place in baking dish and bake for 25 minutes.

PASTA AND TURKEY MEAT RED SAUCE

3 to 4 servings (VITAMIN K content = 12 mcg per cup of sauce. The pasta contains insignificant amounts of vitamin K.)

2	cups	Ground turkey
28	ounces	Canned tomatoes, chopped
1	cup	Finely chopped green pepper
1	cup	Finely chopped onion
2	cloves	Minced garlic
1/2	teaspoon	Fresh oregano, chopped
1/2	teaspoon	Fresh basil, chopped
1 to 2	cups	Plain pasta
1	teaspoon	Olive oil, treated (See DIETARY TIP # 10.)

Cook turkey in olive oil. Drain and throw away fat. Add remaining ingredients, except pasta, and bring to a boil. Cook on low heat for at least one hour.

Cook desired amount of plain pasta. Serve sauce over pasta.

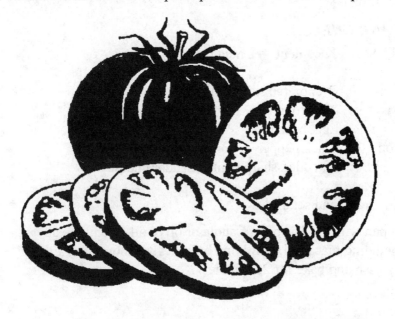

MEAT PASTA SAUCE

6 servings (11 mcgs of vitamin K per serving.)

1/4	cup	Extra-virgin olive oil, treated (See TIP # 10)
1/2	cup	Carrot, diced
1/2	cup	Onion, diced
1/2	cup	Celery stalk, diced
1	large	Garlic clove, minced
1	pound	Italian sausage
1/3	pound	Ground beef
6 1/2	ounces	Pancetta, diced (found in Italian stores, Prosciutto would be a good substitute if you can not find Pancetta)
1/2	teaspoon	Salt
1/2	teaspoon	Freshly ground pepper
1/4	teaspoon	Freshly grated nutmeg
1/2	cup	Dry red wine
3/4	cup	Tomato puree
1	cup	Italian tomatoes, chopped
1/2	ounce	Dried porcini mushrooms (soaked in warm water for at least 1/2 hour)

Remove the Porcini from the water, squeeze dry and finely chop.

Meanwhile, in a large saucepan or flameproof casserole, heat the olive oil over moderate heat. Add the carrot, onion and celery and sauté until the onion is golden, about 4 minutes. Add the garlic and cook until fragrant, about 1 minute. Add the sausage, ground beef and pancetta to the pan. Cook over moderate heat, stirring to break up the meat, until the beef and sausage are no longer pink. Drain off any fat. Season with the salt, pepper and nutmeg.

Pour in the red wine and cook, stirring occasionally, until it evaporates, about 5 minutes. Add the tomato puree, tomatoes, porcini and 1/4 cup of warm water. Simmer for 30 minutes. If the sauce gets too thick, add a little more water. Serve hot over polenta or pasta.

(This can be made up to 2 days ahead. Cover and refrigerate. Reheat before serving.)

MY RICE-A-RONI

6 servings (4 mcgs of vitamin K per serving.)

1/2	cup	Rice (wild)
1	cup	Rice (white)
1	cup	Vermicelli
3	cups	Chicken broth
1/4	cup	Onion
1	clove	Garlic
1	cup	Mushrooms
3/4	cup	Bell pepper
3	tablespoons	Parmesan cheese (or more according to your taste.)
2	tablespoons	Oil, olive or Canola, treated (See DIETARY TIP # 10.)
1	tablespoon	Butter

Sauté onion and green pepper in butter and oil. Add white rice and vermicelli and brown. Add the rest of the ingredients. Bring to a boil, reduce heat and simmer for 30 to 35 minutes. Periodically check the water level and add more if necessary.

Serve hot. Add the parmesan just before serving.

MICROWAVE DIRECTIONS: After you bring the mixture to a boil, put in the microwave on full power for 13 minutes. Check the liquid level and rice for doneness. Add more liquid if necessary and cook on full power for another 5 minutes if necessary.

QUICK TOMATO SAUCE FOR PASTA

8 servings (38 mcgs of vitamin K per serving.)

3/4	cup	Onion, finely chopped
5	cloves	Garlic, crushed
10	tablespoons	Olive oil, treated (See DIETARY TIP # 10.)
28	ounces	Italian-style tomatoes, cut in small pieces
1	ounce	Fresh basil
2	teaspoons	Salt and pepper to taste
1	tablespoon	Sugar

To make sauce, sauté onion and garlic in olive oil until golden. Add undrained tomatoes, basil and 2 teaspoons salt. Season with pepper to taste. Bring to boil and simmer 15 minutes. Add sugar at last minute. Serve over pasta or polenta.

POLENTA

4 servings (Less than 7 mcgs of vitamin K per serving.)

1	cup	Corn meal
1	cup	Cold water
3	cups	Boiling water
		Salt to taste (approximately 1/2 teaspoon)
2	tablespoons	Butter
1/4	cup	Parmesan cheese

Mix the corn meal and salt with the cup of cold water. Slowly whisk this mixture into the boiling water. Reduce heat to medium.

Cook for about 15 minutes, stirring frequently.

Mix in butter and cheese. Pour into serving dish. Serve hot with your favorite Italian sauce.

You can make this ahead and reheat in a microwave or regular oven.

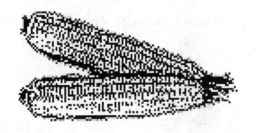

SHRIMP AND WINE-SAUCED SPAGHETTI

2 servings (18 mcgs of vitamin K per serving.)

2	teaspoons	Olive oil, treated (See DIETARY TIP # 10.)
2		Green onions, chopped (about 1/4 cup)
1	clove	Garlic, minced
3	cups	Tomatoes, not drained
2	tablespoons	White wine
1	teaspoon	Sugar
1	teaspoon	Basil, fresh
1/4	teaspoon	Oregano, fresh
1	dash	Pepper, black
8	ounces	Shrimp, peeled and cleaned (You could substitute chicken breast)
1	tablespoon	Cornstarch
1	tablespoon	Cold water
4	ounces	Spaghetti, hot
1	tablespoon	Romano cheese, grated

Sauté onion and garlic in oil. Add undrained tomatoes, wine, sugar and seasonings. Cover, simmer 25 minutes. Add shrimp (or chicken), return to simmer and cook about 5 minutes until tender (if using chicken cook a little longer).

Blend cornstarch in 1 tablespoon cold water, stir into shrimp mixture. Cook until bubbly. Serve over the hot spaghetti and sprinkle with cheese.

Serve immediately. This is wonderful with a good French bread.

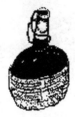

PASTA JAMBALAYA

4 servings (33 mcgs of vitamin K per serving.)

2	teaspoons	Olive oil, treated (See DIETARY TIP # 10.)
8	ounces	Hot Italian turkey sausage, cut in 1 inch pieces
8	ounces	Boneless skinless chicken breasts cut in 1 inch pieces
1/2	pound	Shrimp, medium, shelled and deveined
2	cups	Green bell peppers cut in strips
1	cup	Chopped onion
3	cloves	Garlic, minced
2	cups	Canned crushed tomatoes (or Italian tomatoes)
1/2	cup	Clam juice
1/4	cup	Chicken broth
1/2	teaspoon	Basil, fresh
1/4	teaspoon	Garlic powder
1/4	teaspoon	Salt
1/8	teaspoon	Ground red pepper
6	ounces	Fresh or dried fettuccine

In a large non-stick skillet, heat the oil. Add sausage, cook, stir often, 6-8 minutes or until brown. Add chicken, cook, stirring often for 5 minutes. Add shrimp, cook 3 minutes longer or until chicken is brown and shrimp is pink. Move meat to a plate.

Add green peppers, onions and garlic to skillet, cook, stirring often, 3 minutes or until tender. Add tomatoes and remaining ingredients except pasta. Bring to boil and add the meat back to the pan. Reduce to low and simmer 15 minutes.

Meanwhile cook pasta, drain, add to skillet, toss and serve.

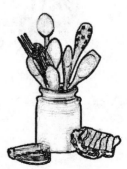

POLISH NOODLES AND CABBAGE

4 servings (90 mcgs of vitamin K per serving.)

1/4	cup	Butter
1/2	cup	Onion, chopped
1/2	pound	Cabbage, sliced thin
1	teaspoon	Caraway seeds or fennel seed
8	ounces	Egg noodles
1/2	cup	Sour cream
1/8	teaspoon	Black pepper, freshly ground
1/2	teaspoon	Salt

Melt the butter in a large skillet. Add the onion and sauté until transparent. Add the cabbage and sauté 5 minutes or until tender but still crisp. Stir in the caraway seeds, salt and pepper.

Meanwhile, cook the noodles in salted water as directed on package. Do not overcook. Drain well.

Stir the noodles into the cabbage and add the sour cream. Cook 5 minutes longer, stirring frequently.

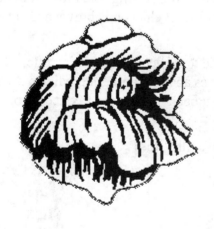

HERBED RICE TOSS

4 servings (6 mcgs of vitamin K per serving.)

2	tablespoons	Plus 2 teaspoon butter
1/2	cup	Chopped onions
1	clove	Garlic, minced
1	cup	Chopped celery
2	cups	Chopped mushrooms
1/2	teaspoon	Sage, fresh, chopped
1/2	teaspoon	Thyme, fresh, chopped
1	packet	Instant chicken-broth mix (or 1 bouillon cube)
2	cups	Cooked brown rice

Melt butter in a large nonstick skillet over medium heat. Add onions, garlic, and celery. Sauté until tender, about 10 minutes.

Add mushrooms, spices, and broth mix. Cook, stirring occasionally, 10 more minutes, until mushrooms are tender. Add small amounts of water, if necessary to prevent drying.

Add rice. Toss until heated through.

This goes especially well with baked chicken or fish.

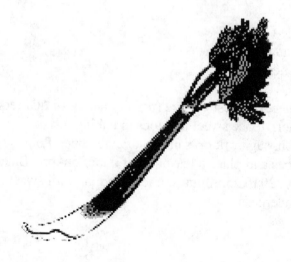

CHEESY RICE AND HAM

4 servings (13 mcgs of vitamin K per serving.)

1 /12	cups	CHEDDAR CHEESE SAUCE (See Recipe Index.)
2	cups	Rice, cooked
2	cups	Ham, diced
1	cup	Corn, drained
1	cup	Colby cheese, shredded
1/2	cup	Green onion, chopped

In a large bowl, combine soup, milk, and stir to blend. Add rice, ham and corn. Turn mix into a 10 by 6 inch baking pan. Sprinkle with cheese. Bake at 350 degrees Fahrenheit for 30 minutes. MICROWAVE: Cook on HIGH for 7-10 minutes, or until heated through, stirring once. Then top with shredded cheese and cook on HIGH for 2 minutes or until cheese is melted.

CANDIED SWEET POTATOES

6 servings (VITAMIN K content = 10 mcg per cup)

3	cups	Skinless sweet potatoes
1	teaspoon	Ground cinnamon
1/2	cup	Brown sugar
2	teaspoons	Flour
1/2	teaspoon	Salt
1	cup	Orange juice
		Butter

Cut sweet potatoes into pieces of desired size (usually halves or quarters) and boil until mildly tender. Place sweet potatoes in baking dish. Mix together the cinnamon, sugar, flour, salt and orange juice. Pour mixture over sweet potatoes and place a teaspoon of butter on top. Bake at 350 degrees Fahrenheit for 20 to 25 minutes, uncovered, or until sweet potatoes are at desired tenderness.

LEMON HERB ROASTED POTATOES

6 servings (15 mcgs of vitamin K per serving.)

2 1/2	pounds	Small red potatoes
1/4	cup	Olive oil, treated (See DIETARY TIP # 10.)
2	tablespoons	Lemon juice, fresh
1	teaspoon	Salt
1	teaspoon	Fresh oregano
1	teaspoon	Fresh thyme
1/4	teaspoon	Paprika
1/4	teaspoon	Pepper, finely ground

Preheat the oven to 425 degrees Fahrenheit. Wash the potatoes, rinse, and pat dry. Cut each into 3/4 inch dice.

Combine the olive oil, lemon juice, salt, oregano, thyme, paprika, and pepper in a large bowl and mix well. Add the potatoes and toss.

Arrange the potatoes on an oiled baking sheet and bake about 35 minutes, turning every 15 minutes, until tender and well browned. Taste for seasoning.

Turn into a serving dish and serve immediately.

ADVANCE PREPARATION: This may be prepared 2 hours in advance and kept at room temperature. Reheat in a 350 degree Fahrenheit oven for 10 to 15 minutes. Serve with scrambled eggs, omelets, sautéed chicken or grilled veal chops.

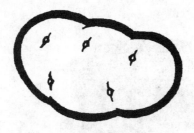

POTATO CASSEROLE

6 servings (5 mcgs of vitamin K per serving.)

8	large	Potatoes, cooked
1	can	Cream of chicken or cream of mushroom soup
2	cups	Green beans, cooked
1/2	cup	Chopped onion
1/2	cup	Green pepper, chopped
1 1/2	cups	Shredded Cheddar cheese
2	tablespoons	Olive oil, treated (See DIETARY TIP # 10.)
1/2	teaspoon	Rosemary, ground
		Crushed corn flakes or bread crumbs

Sauté onion and green pepper in olive oil.

Peel and slice (or dice) potatoes. Blend with soup, green beans and grated cheese. Place in a 2-1/2 quart oiled baking dish. Sprinkle corn flakes or bread crumbs on top of the casserole.

Bake in a preheated 350 degree Fahrenheit oven for 45 minutes to an hour, until all bubbly and potatoes are tender.

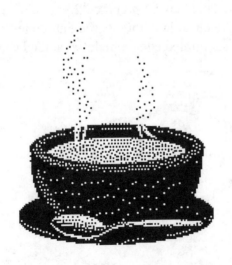

VEGETABLES

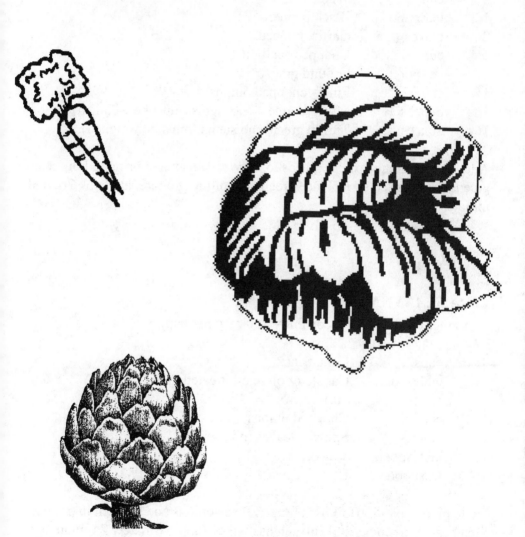

SMOTHERED GREENS

4 servings (VITAMIN K content = 400 mcg per cup)

2	slices	Bacon
3	cups	Water
1/2	teaspoon	Black pepper
2	cloves	Garlic, minced
1/4	cup	Chopped scallion
1	teaspoon	Ground ginger
1/4	cup	Finely chopped onions
16	ounces	Mustard greens, no stems (must be weighed)
16	ounces	Turnip greens, no stems (must be weighed)

Add all ingredients except greens to large saucepan and bring to boil. Cut greens into desired size. Place greens in boiling mixture and cook 20 to 30 minutes.

LIMA BEANS AND SPINACH

8 servings (VITAMIN K content = 260 mcg per cup)

4	cups	Lima beans
1	tablespoon	Canola or olive oil, treated (See DIETARY TIP # 10.)
1	cup	Chopped onions
16	ounces	Spinach leaves (no stems)
1	tablespoon	Vinegar
1/4	teaspoon	Black pepper

Sauté onions in oil. Boil lima beans. Place onions and spinach in pot with lima beans and cook until spinach has wilted (approximately 2 minutes). Add vinegar and pepper.

VEGETABLE STEW

12 servings (VITAMIN K content = 35 mcg per cup)

3	cups	Water
2	cups	Skinned, chopped potatoes
2	cups	Chopped carrots
4	cups	Chopped squash
2	cups	Sweet corn
2	cloves	Garlic, minced
1/2	cup	Chopped scallions
1/4	cup	Chopped green pepper
1	cup	Chopped onion
1	cup	Chopped tomatoes

Bring water to boil. Add carrots and potatoes. Cook for 10 minutes on low boil. Add remaining ingredients except tomatoes and cook for 15 more minutes. Add tomatoes and cook for 5 more minutes.

SUCCOTASH

6 servings (7 mcgs of vitamin K per serving.)

1/4	cup	Ham, diced
1	pound	Fresh or frozen lima beans
3	cups	Fresh or frozen corn
1/2	teaspoon	Salt
	dash	Pepper
1/3	cup	Water
1/4	cup	Milk

Brown the ham in the pan. Add all ingredients except milk. Bring to a boil. Turn down heat to simmer. Cook for 20 to 25 minutes until the lima beans are tender. Add milk and heat but do not boil.

MAPLE WHIPPED BUTTERNUT SQUASH

7 to 8 servings (5 mcgs of vitamin K per serving.)

2	pounds	Butternut squash, peeled, quartered and seeded
1/2	cup	Butter, softened
1/4	cup	Maple syrup
1	tablespoon	Light brown sugar, firmly packed
1/4	teaspoon	Nutmeg, freshly grated
		Salt and freshly grated white pepper, to taste

Bring 1 1/2 inches water to boil in 5-quart sauce pot or Dutch oven. Add squash and steam, covered, until tender, about 20 minutes. Drain, then return to pot and mash and stir over low heat about 5 minutes to evaporate some of moisture.

Transfer to large bowl and add butter, maple syrup, brown sugar, salt and pepper. Beat with electric mixer at medium speed, or with potato masher, until smooth. Sprinkle with nutmeg to serve.

STUFFED ARTICHOKES

4 servings (13 mcgs of vitamin K per serving.)

4		Artichokes
2	cups	Bread crumbs
1	cup	Parmesan cheese
2	clove	Garlic, minced
		Salt and pepper
1/4	cup	Olive oil, treated (See DIETARY TIP # 10.)

Cut off the artichoke stems very evenly so they stand up alone. Cut off the top fourth of the artichoke leaves. Spread the leaves so they resemble a rose and wash them. Turn the artichokes upside down to dry.

In a bowl, mix the remaining ingredients except the olive oil. Pour a little olive oil over the mixture to make a paste.

Put some of the paste mixture in between every leaf and layer of the artichokes.

With a little water at the bottom of a large pot, steam the artichokes for approximately 1 hour. Add additional water as it evaporates. Serve warm or at room temperature.

BALSAMIC SQUASH PUREE

4 servings (4 mcgs of vitamin K per serving.)

2	tablespoons	Shallots, minced
1/4	cup	Butter
3	tablespoons	Balsamic vinegar
2	cups	Roast squash pulp
1	teaspoon	Salt
		Freshly grated nutmeg

Cook shallots in a medium saucepan with 1 tablespoon of butter over medium heat until soft, about 3 to 5 minutes.

Add vinegar, increase heat to high, and cook until vinegar is reduced to syrup, another 3 to 5 minutes.

Add squash pulp and salt and stir to combine. Reduce heat to low and cook until heated through, about 5 minutes.

Cut remaining butter into small cubes, add to squash, and beat in until fairly smooth. Serve immediately, dusted with freshly grated nutmeg.

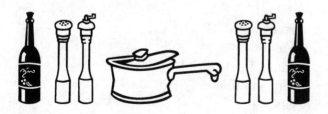

SUMMER SQUASH STIR-FRY

6 servings (5 mcgs of vitamin K per serving.)

2	tablespoons	Olive oil, treated (See DIETARY TIP # 10.)
1	clove	Garlic, minced
3/4	cup	Onion, sliced and separated into rings
3	medium	Zucchini, peeled, thinly sliced or julienne
3	medium	Yellow squash, peeled, thinly sliced
8		Cherry tomatoes, cut in half or 2 tomatoes cut in 1/2 inch pieces
1/2	teaspoon	Salt
1/2	teaspoon	Pepper
1/4	cup	Grated Parmesan cheese

Pour 2 tablespoons oil around top of preheated wok, coating sides. Heat at medium high (325 degrees Fahrenheit) for 1 minute.

Add garlic clove and onion, stir-fry 1 minute.

Add zucchini and yellow squash, stir-fry 3 minutes or until crisp-tender.

Add cherry tomatoes, salt, and pepper, stir-fry 1 minute or until thoroughly heated.

Transfer to a serving bowl. Sprinkle with cheese, and serve immediately.

STRING BEANS, SOUTHERN STYLE

4 servings (1 mcgs of vitamin K per serving.)

1	pound	Green beans
1/2	cup	Water
3/4	cup	Onion, finely diced
1/3	cup	Ham, cut fine
1/4	teaspoon	Salt
	dash	Pepper
1/8	teaspoon	Paprika

Wash beans, cut slantwise into 1-inch lengths, add water, onion, ham and seasonings. Bring to a boil. Turn down heat to a simmer, cover pan and cook for 25 to 30 minutes until beans are tender and juices are reduced to one half.

FRIED GARLIC GREEN BEANS

4 servings (9 mcgs of vitamin K per serving.)

1	pound	Fresh green beans, cleaned
6-10	cloves	Garlic, minced
1	tablespoon	Olive oil, treated (See DIETARY TIP # 10.)
1/4	teaspoon	White pepper
1/4	teaspoon	Salt (optional)

Steam the green beans until almost done. Try to time the steaming so that the green beans are ready at the same time as the garlic is ready in the next step.

Heat the olive oil in a skillet large enough to toss stuff about in without getting it all over the place. Add the garlic and sauté until it just begins to turn brown.

Add the green beans to the skillet along with the pepper and salt and toss to coat with the oil and garlic.

Raise the heat a little and toss continuously until the green beans start to get brown and black in some spots. Then remove from the skillet into your serving dish. Serve hot.

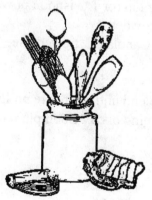

BABY CARROTS GLAZED WITH BUTTER

4 servings (9 mcgs of vitamin K per serving.)

2	pounds	Baby carrots, scraped (they usually come already scraped these days)
3	tablespoons	Butter
		Salt and freshly ground black pepper

Place the carrots in a heavy saucepan and barely cover with water. Add the butter and cover.

Bring to a boil, reduce the heat, and cook 15 minutes or until still firm but easy to pierce with a fork.

Remove the cover and boil down until the liquid has evaporated and the carrots are coated with butter. Watch them carefully or they will burn. Season with salt and pepper.

CAULIFLOWER PANCAKES

6 servings (4 mcgs of vitamin K per serving.)

1 1/4	cups	Cauliflower, cut in small pieces
1/2	tablespoon	Flour
1	large	Egg
1/2	teaspoon	Salt
2	teaspoons	Grated onion (or 1 teaspoon powdered onion)
1/2	teaspoon	Baking powder
1/2	cup	Olive or Canola oil, treated (See TIP # 10) for frying

Put everything in blender and blend until there are no lumps. Make small 2 inch pancakes. Fry in oil, turning once. Good plain or with sour cream.

ZUCCHINI AND CHEDDAR BAKE

8 servings (4 mcgs of vitamin K per serving.)

| 4 | cups | Zucchini, peeled and coarsely grated |
| 1/2 | pound | Grated cheddar cheese |

Layer 1/3 zucchini, 1/3 cheese, salt and pepper to taste. Repeat. Bake at 350 degrees Fahrenheit for 40 minutes.

CAULIFLOWER WITH TOMATOES

6 servings (12 mcgs of vitamin K per serving.)

4	cups	Fresh cauliflower in bite size pieces
1/2	cup	Water
1/2	teaspoon	Oregano
1/4	teaspoon	Salt
2	medium	Tomatoes, in wedges
1/2	cup	Mozzarella cheese, shredded

Place cauliflower and water in a 2-quart dish, cover. Microwave on HIGH for 5 to 8 minutes or until tender-crisp. Drain.

Stir in seasonings and tomatoes. Microwave uncovered, at HIGH 2 to 4 minutes, or until tomatoes are hot. Sprinkle with Mozzarella cheese. Microwave 1 minute or until cheese melts.

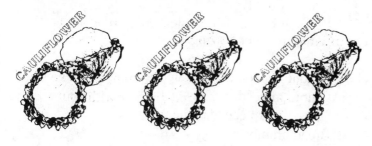

STUFFED PEPPERS

6 servings (37 mcgs of vitamin K per serving.)

6		Green peppers (about 2 1/2 pounds)
1	pound	Ground beef
1	cup	Cooked rice
16	ounces	Tomato sauce
1/4	teaspoon	Black pepper
1	clove	Garlic, minced
2	tablespoons	Chopped onion (not green onion or scallions)
1	quart	Water

Cut a slice in stem end of peppers. Remove seeds and thoroughly wash. Bring 3/4 cup water per pepper to boil, add peppers and cook for 5 minutes. Remove peppers. Preheat oven to 350 degrees Fahrenheit.

Cook beef, garlic and onion in skillet until onion is tender. Drain off fat and stir in rice, and half the tomato sauce. Heat mixture. Stuff each pepper and stand upright in baking dish. Pour rest of tomato sauce over peppers and bake, covered, 45 minutes. Uncover and bake 15 minutes.

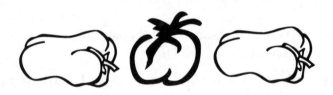

ZUCCHINI CASSEROLE

4 servings (10 mcgs of vitamin K per serving.)

1	pound	Zucchini, peeled and grated
1/3	cup	Onion, minced
1	cup	Grated sharp cheddar cheese
1	cup	Bread crumbs
2		Eggs, beaten
3	tablespoons	Melted butter
1/2	teaspoon	Salt
1/4	teaspoon	Pepper

HERB MIXTURE

1/4	cup	Celery leaves chopped
1	teaspoon	Mixed fresh herbs, like thyme, sage and marjoram

Drain the zucchini. Combine the zucchini, onion, cheese, bread crumbs, eggs, butter, salt and pepper.

For herb mixture, chop the celery leaves together with the fresh herbs to freshen the flavor. Stir into the zucchini mixture.

Spoon mixture into a buttered 9-inch pie plate. Bake at 350 degrees Fahrenheit for 40-45 minutes or until golden.

Let cool for about 10 minutes before serving.

ZUCCHINI-TOMATO PIE

6 servings (7 mcgs of vitamin K per serving.)

2	cups	Zucchini, peeled and chopped
1	cup	Tomato, chopped
1/2	cup	Onion, chopped
1/3	cup	Parmesan cheese, grated
1 1/2	cups	Milk
3/4	cup	Bisquick baking mix, low-fat
3		Eggs
1/2	teaspoon	Salt
1/4	teaspoon	Pepper

Heat oven to 400 degrees Fahrenheit. Grease 10 inch quiche dish or pie plate, 10 by 1 1/2 inches.

Sprinkle zucchini, tomato, onion and cheese in plate. Beat remaining ingredients until smooth, 15 seconds in blender on high or 1 minute with hand beater. Pour into plate.

Bake until knife inserted in center comes out clean, about 30 minutes. Cool 5 minutes.

BASQUE PEPPER STEW

4 servings (28 mcgs of vitamin K per serving.)

2	tablespoons	Olive or Canola oil, treated (See DIETARY TIP # 10.)
1	cup	Onion, chopped
2 to 3		Green peppers (1 pound), cored, seeded, cut into 1/4 by 1/2 inch cubes.
2	cloves	Garlic, chopped
1 1/2	pounds	Ripe tomatoes, peeled, seeded and chopped.
		Salt and fresh ground pepper to taste

Heat oil in deep skillet over low heat. Add onion and cook, stirring often, until soft but not brown, about 5 minutes. Add green peppers and garlic and cook, stirring often, until peppers soften, about 7 minutes. Add tomatoes and salt and pepper to taste. Cook, uncovered, over medium heat, stirring often, until stew is thick, about 30 minutes. Taste and adjust seasoning.

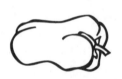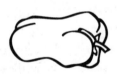

BEST EVER BAKED BEANS

12 servings (4 mcgs of vitamin K per serving.)

4 1/2	pounds	Canned pork and beans
1/2	cup	Onion, chopped
1/2	cup	Celery, chopped
1/3	cup	Bell pepper, chopped
2	tablespoons	Prepared mustard
1/2	cup	Molasses
1	teaspoon	Worcestershire sauce
4	drops	Tabasco sauce

1/2	cup	Barbecue sauce
1/2	cup	Catsup
2	Strips	Bacon, uncooked, and cut in half

Combine all ingredients, except bacon, in a large oven-proof container. Lay bacon strips on top. Place on a smoker barbecue grid and smoke-cook for 2 to 2 1/2 hours. (Or put them in your oven at 325 degrees Fahrenheit for 2 1/2 hours.)

ONION PANCAKES

6 servings (2 mcgs of vitamin K per serving.)

1	pound	Plain flour
8	ounces	Boiling water
1/2	pint	Cold water
1	pound	Onions, peeled and finely chopped
5	tablespoons	Canola or olive oil, treated (See DIETARY TIP # 10.)
1 1/2	tablespoons	Salt

Sift the flour into a bowl. Pour in the boiling water, stirring all the time to form a stiff dough. Add the cold water to the dough and when it is cool enough to handle, knead until smooth. Cover the dough and leave to rest for about 30 minutes.

Roll the dough into a long sausage and cut into 10 pieces. Roll each piece into a ball, then flatten with the rolling pin into a small pancake about 3 to 4 inches in diameter. Sprinkle each pancake with the chopped onion and salt. Fold the edges of the pancake into the middle and then roll out into a pancake again.

Heat 2 tablespoons of vegetable oil in a frying pan and put in the pancakes. Fry in batches for 2 minutes on either side, or until golden brown, adding more oil as necessary.

Serve hot either by themselves or as an accompaniment to savory foods.

LEMON VEGGIES

4 servings (VITAMIN K content = 165 mcg per cup) Be careful with serving this recipe! Make certain there are approximately equal amounts of all vegetables! Also, you must weigh the broccoli, not just measure the amount in a measuring cup.)

1	cup	Raw cauliflower
1	cup	Raw broccoli (weight = 8 ounces)
1	cup	Raw carrots
3	tablespoons	Lemon juice
1	tablespoon	Olive or Canola oil, treated (See DIETARY TIP # 10.)
1	clove	Garlic, minced

Steam vegetables until tender. Mix remaining ingredients in saucepan and cook over low heat for 3 minutes. Pour sauce over vegetables in serving dish.

PINEAPPLE YAM BAKE

6 servings (5 mcgs of vitamin K per serving.)

3	medium	Yams, about 1 1/2 pounds, sliced 1 inch thick
3/4	cup	Crushed pineapple, juice pack, drained
4	tablespoons	Pure maple syrup
2		Egg whites

Cook yams in boiling water for 25 to 35 minutes or until very soft and tender. Drain and mash thoroughly until consistency is smooth. Preheat oven to 400 degrees Fahrenheit. Mix drained pineapple and 3 tablespoons syrup into mashed yams. Spoon into a 9 inch round or 8 inch square non-stick baking pan. Beat egg whites to soft peaks, add remaining 1 tablespoon syrup and beat until stiff. Spread with a spatula, using a swirling motion, on top of yam mixture. Bake at 400 degrees Fahrenheit for 8 to 10 minutes, or until top is golden.

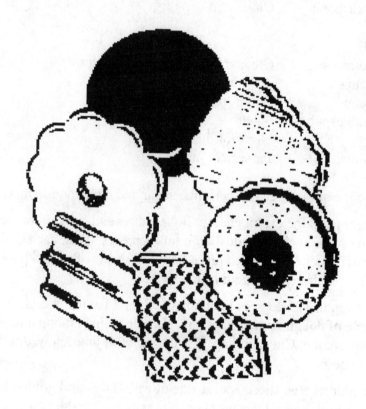

COOKIES

RUGALA

48 servings (1 mcg of VITAMIN K per serving.)

FILLING:

1	cup	Ground pecans
1	cup	Raisins
1/2	cup	Sugar
1	teaspoon	Cinnamon

DOUGH:

8	ounces	Cream cheese, room temperature
2	cups	All purpose flour
1	cup	Butter, room temperature
2	tablespoons	Sugar
		Flour for dusting
12	ounces	Jar apricot jam

For filling: combine pecans, currants, sugar and cinnamon in mixing bowl.

For dough: combine cream cheese, flour, butter and sugar in processor or mixer and blend well. Divide dough into 4 pieces. Dust each with flour, shaking off excess. Roll each piece between sheets of waxed paper into 10 inch circle. Refrigerate 1 hour or longer

Preheat oven to 375 degrees Fahrenheit. Grease baking sheets. Spread each circle of dough with apricot jam. Divide filling among circles, spreading evenly. Cut each into 12 wedges. Roll up each wedge from bottom to point.

Arrange on prepared sheets, point side down. Bake until golden brown, about 16-17 minutes. Transfer at once to wire rack and let cool.

Store cookies in airtight container.

Tips: Be sure to work on just one circle at a time and keep the others refrigerated. Do not overdo the jam and cinnamon and pecan filling because they tend to overflow and will burn on your baking sheets.

PUMPKIN BARS WITH CREAM CHEESE FROSTING
40 servings (1 mcg of VITAMIN K per serving.)

2	cups	Sugar
8	ounces	Pumpkin and/or papaya
2	cups	Bisquick or similar mix, low-fat
1/2	cup	Raisins
1/2	cup	Cottage cheese
4	large	Eggs or 1 cup of an egg substitute
2	tablespoons	Cinnamon
		CREAM CHEESE FROSTING (See Recipe Index for recipe.)

Preheat oven to 350 degrees Fahrenheit.

Grease a jelly roll pan, 15 1/2 by 10 1/2 by 1 inch size.

Beat sugar, oil, pumpkin and eggs on medium speed in mixer for one minute.

Stir in Bisquick, cinnamon and raisins. Pour into prepared pan. Bake until toothpick inserted in center comes out clean, about 25 to 30 minutes. Cool. Frost and cut into 3 inch by 1 inch bars.

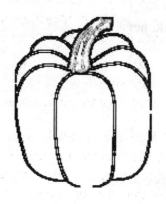

CREAM CHEESE FROSTING

Yields enough to frost two 9 inch layers. (VITAMIN K content = 9 mcg for the entire recipe)

3	ounces	Cream cheese, softened (may use lite cream cheese)
1/3	cup	Butter
2	cups	Powdered sugar, sifted
1	tablespoon	Milk
1	teaspoon	Vanilla

Beat cream cheese, butter, milk and vanilla until creamy. Stir in confectioners sugar and beat until smooth.

MEXICAN WEDDING COOKIES

36 servings (1 mcg of VITAMIN K per serving.)

1	cup	Butter, softened
1	cup	Powdered sugar
2	cups	Sifted flour
1	cup	Ground nuts
1	teaspoon	Vanilla

Combine all ingredients.

Form into 1 1/2 inch balls.

Bake on cookie sheet at 350 degrees Fahrenheit for about 10-15 minutes or until set.

Roll in powdered sugar while still warm.

CHOCOLATE WALNUT SQUARES

24 servings (1 mcg of VITAMIN K per serving.)

1 1/4	cups	Sifted all-purpose flour
3/4	cup	Brown sugar, packed
1		Egg, large
3/4	teaspoon	Baking powder
1/4	cup	Coffee liqueur
1/2	teaspoon	Salt
1	cup	Semi-sweet chocolate pieces
1/2	cup	Soft butter
1/3	cup	Chopped walnuts
1	tablespoon	Coffee liqueur for tops of bars
		BROWN BUTTER ICING (See Recipe Index)

Resift flour with baking powder and salt.

Cream butter, sugar and egg together well.

Stir in coffee liqueur, then flour mixture, blending well. Fold in chocolate pieces and walnuts. Spread evenly in greased baking pan 7 by 11 by 1 1/2-inches.

Bake in 350 degrees Fahrenheit oven, 30 minutes or until top springs back when touched lightly in the center. Remove from oven, cool in pan, for 15 minutes. Then brush top with remaining tablespoon of coffee liqueur. When cold, spread with BROWN BUTTER ICING. When icing is set, cut into bars about 1 3/4 by 1 1/2 inches. Makes 2 dozen.

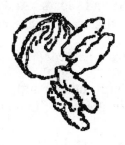

BROWN BUTTER ICING
1 recipe (VITAMIN K content = 2 mcg for the entire recipe)

2	tablespoons	Butter
1	tablespoon	Coffee liqueur
2	teaspoons	Milk or light cream
1/3	cup	Powdered sugar, sifted

Place 2 tablespoons butter in saucepan over low heat. Heat until lightly browned. Remove and add 1 tablespoon coffee liqueur, 2 teaspoons milk or light cream, and 1/3 cup sifted powdered sugar. Beat smooth. (You may need to add a little more sugar to the icing.) Use as directed in recipe.

PEANUT BUTTER COOKIES
50 servings (1 mcg of VITAMIN K per serving.)

1	teaspoon	Vanilla
1	cup	Sugar
1	cup	Brown sugar
1	cup	Butter
2		Egg
1	cup	Peanut butter
3	cups	Flour
1/8	teaspoon	Salt
2	teaspoons	Baking soda

Cream together shortening, vanilla and sugars. Add eggs. Mix together the dry ingredients and add to the first mixture and mix well. It will be dry at first.

Form into small balls and place on greased cookie sheet. Press with a fork that has been dipped in sugar (to prevent sticking). Press to make a criss cross pattern. They will remain the same size in diameter, so what you see is what you get.

Bake at 375 degrees Fahrenheit for 10 minutes.

FUDGE BROWNIES

12 servings (VITAMIN K content = 3 mcg per serving)

1/2	cup	Butter
2	ounces	Unsweetened chocolate
1	cup	Sugar
2	large	Eggs
1	tablespoon	Vanilla
3/4	cup	Flour
1/2	cup	Walnuts, chopped
		CHOCOLATE FROSTING (See Recipe Index.)

Preheat oven to 350 degrees Fahrenheit. Grease an 8 by 8 inch baking pan.

Melt butter and chocolate. Remove from heat and stir in the sugar. Add eggs and vanilla, beat lightly just until blended. Stir in flour and nuts. Spread batter in pan.

Bake 30 minutes. Cool. Ice with CHOCOLATE FROSTING (See Recipe Index for Frosting recipe.) and cut into bars.

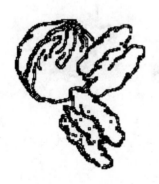

CHOCOLATE FROSTING:

2 cups (VITAMIN K content = 3 mcg per recipe)

1	cup	Sugar
3	tablespoons	Butter
2	ounces	Unsweetened chocolate
1/4	cup	Milk
3	cups	Confectioners sugar, sifted

Melt butter, add chocolate and stir until chocolate melts. Remove from heat and stir in sugar. Add milk and put back on burner. Cook, stirring constantly until mixture is bubbly. Cool a little before using. Use as directed in recipe.

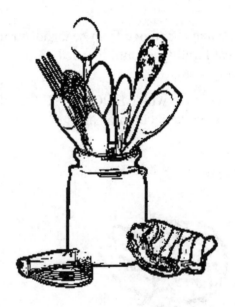

RAISIN-FILLED BARS

27 servings (2 mcgs of VITAMIN K per serving.)

FILLING

2	cups	Raisins
1 1/3	cups	Water
3	tablespoons	Cornstarch
2	tablespoons	Cold water
1	cup	Sugar
1	teaspoon	Vanilla

COOKIE

1	cup	Brown sugar, firmly packed
1 1/2	cups	Rolled oats
1	cup	Melted butter
1 1/2	cups	Sifted flour
1	teaspoon	Baking soda
1/2	teaspoon	Salt
1	cup	Chopped nuts

FILLING: Cook raisins in 1 1/3 cup water until tender. Dissolve cornstarch in 2 tablespoon cold water. Add sugar and cornstarch to raisins, stir until mix thickens. Remove from heat, add vanilla and set aside to cool.

COOKIE: Add brown sugar and oats to melted butter. Mix well.

Sift together flour, soda and salt. Add to sugar and butter mixture. Stir in nuts. Pack half of mix into bottom of 9 inch square pan. Spread raisin filling evenly on top. Top with remaining crumb mixture.

Bake in 350 degrees Fahrenheit oven for 30 minutes. Set pan on rack to cool 10 minutes, or cool completely, then cut in 3 by 1 inch bars.

ALMOND BUTTER COOKIES

36 cookies (1 mcg of VITAMIN K per 3 cookies)

1	cup	Butter
1	teaspoon	Almond extract
1/4	teaspoon	Salt
2	cups	Flour
1/2	cup	Sugar

Cream butter and sugar with extract. Add salt and flour. Mix well. Chill dough. Form into 1 inch balls and roll in sugar. Stamp each cookie with cookie stamp. Bake at 350 degrees 12 to 15 minutes.

SOUR CREAM COOKIES

36 cookies (1 mcg of VITAMIN K per 3 cookies)

1/2	cup	Butter
1	large	Egg
1/2	cup	Sour cream
2 1/2	cups	Flour (sifted)
1	cup	Sugar
1/2	teaspoon	Baking soda
1/2	teaspoon	Salt
1	teaspoon	Vanilla

Cream together shortening and sugar. Add egg and beat well. Add sour cream. Add flour (sifted), soda and salt. Blend all together and drop onto an ungreased cookie sheet.

Dip the bottom of a small glass in water and then into sugar and press on top of dropped cookie dough, flattening the cookie a bit. Bake 12 to 16 minutes at 335 degrees Fahrenheit.

CAKES

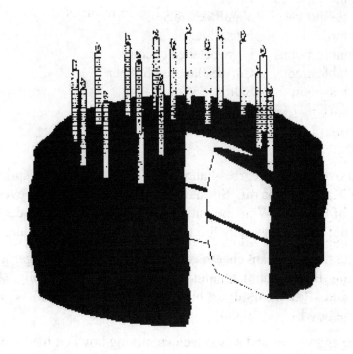

MARBLE CHEESECAKE

10 servings (1 mcg of VITAMIN K per serving. This recipe is also low in fat and calories.)

3		Graham crackers, crushed
15	ounces	Reduced-fat or no-fat ricotta cheese
8	ounces	Reduced-fat cream cheese
1/4	cup	Reduced-fat sour cream
1/2	cup	Sugar, plus
6	tablespoons	Sugar
2	tablespoons	Flour
1 1/2	teaspoons	Vanilla extract
3	large	Egg whites
3	tablespoons	Unsweetened cocoa
1	tablespoon	Coffee-flavored liqueur
1/8	teaspoon	Salt
		Butter or Canola oil for pan
		Boiling water

Preheat oven to 350 degrees Fahrenheit. Grease an 8-inch springform pan with butter or Canola oil. Sprinkle graham cracker crumbs evenly over the bottom of the pan. Wrap the outside of the pan with heavy-duty foil. (If you do not have heavy-duty foil then just double up the regular foil.)

Combine ricotta, cream cheese, sour cream and 1/2 cup sugar in food processor. Process until smooth, scraping sides occasionally. Add flour and vanilla. Process until just blended (about 15 seconds). Transfer batter to a large bowl.

Beat the egg whites and salt in a clean mixing bowl on medium speed until foamy. Gradually beat in remaining 6 tablespoons of sugar, 1 tablespoon at a time. Continue beating until the egg whites form soft peaks.
Carefully fold half the beaten whites into the cheese batter with a rubber spatula. Repeat with the remaining whites.

Transfer 1-1/2 cups of the batter to a medium bowl. Pour the remaining batter over the graham cracker crumbs in the springform pan. Place the foil wrapped springform pan inside a larger baking pan.

Gently whisk the cocoa and liqueur into the reserved batter just until smooth. Carefully spoon the cocoa mixture over the batter in the pan. Swirl a knife through to marbleize.

Place the pans, one inside the other, on the oven rack. Pour boiling water into the larger pan to reach 1 inch up the side of the springform pan. Bake 45 minutes or until just set. Turn the oven off and let the cake stand in the oven for 1 hour with the oven door closed.

Remove the pan from the water bath. Remove foil; cool completely. Cover and refrigerate overnight (or at least 4 to 5 hours). Remove sides of pan, cut and serve.

FRUIT COCKTAIL CAKE
8 servings (1 mcg of VITAMIN K per serving.)

2	cups	Unbleached flour
1 1/2	cups	Sugar
2	cups	Fruit cocktail
2	teaspoons	Baking soda
2	large	Eggs
1/8	teaspoon	Salt

Mix all ingredients in a 9 x 13-inch pan. Mix by hand. Bake at 350 degrees Fahrenheit for about 40 minutes.

CHEESECAKE

10 servings (2 mcgs of VITAMIN K per serving.)

1	tablespoon	Graham cracker crumbs
1	cup	Low fat cottage cheese
16	ounces	Cream cheese*
2/3	cup	Sugar
2	tablespoons	Unbleached all-purpose flour
2	tablespoons	Skim milk
1/4	cup	Almond extract
3	large	Eggs

*Cream Cheese may be Lite and should be softened.

Lightly grease the bottom of a 9-inch springform pan. Sprinkle with crumbs. Remove excess crumbs.

Put cottage cheese in blender container. Cover and process on high speed until smooth. In large mixing bowl of electric mixer, combine cottage cheese, cream cheese, sugar and flour. Mix at medium speed until well blended.

Add eggs, one at a time, mixing well after each addition. Blend in milk and extract, pour into pan.

Bake at 325 degrees Fahrenheit, 45 to 50 minutes or until center is almost set. (Center of cheesecake appears to be soft, but firms upon cooling.)

Cool. Loosen cake from rim of pan and remove rim. Chill.

Top with fresh slices of strawberries or blueberries, if desired. (Adding the fruit will add 1 to 2 mcgs of VITAMIN K per serving.) Macerate strawberries in Cointreau and sugar.

PUMPKIN-RAISIN CAKE

12 servings (3 mcgs of VITAMIN K per serving.)

1 2/3	cups	Flour
2/3	cup	Sugar
1/4	cup	Nonfat dry milk
1	teaspoon	Baking soda
1/2	teaspoon	Baking powder
1/2	teaspoon	Salt
2	teaspoons	Pumpkin pie spice
1/2	cup	Raisins
2		Egg whites
1	cup	Canned pumpkin
1/3	cup	Karo syrup, light or dark
1/3	cup	Orange juice
		Butter for greasing pan

Butter a 9-inch square baking pan.

In large bowl, combine dry ingredients and raisins.

In medium bowl, combine remaining ingredients.

Add to dry ingredients. Stir until smooth. Pour into prepared pan.

Bake in 350 degrees Fahrenheit oven 35 minutes or until toothpick inserted in center comes out clean. Cool in pan on wire rack. (This is a fat free cake but you would not know it!)

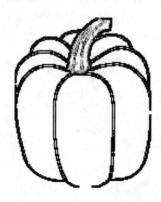

GOLDEN FRUITCAKE

12 servings (4 mcg of VITAMIN K per serving.)

1 1/4	cups	All-purpose flour
1/2	teaspoon	Baking powder
1/2	teaspoon	Salt
2	cups	Candied fruits*
1	cup	Raisins, white
1	cup	Pecans
1/2	cup	Butter
1/2	cup	Sugar
3	large	Eggs
1/2	cup	Bourbon or cognac

*One quarter pound each of candied cherries and small pieces of candied pineapple.

Line a well buttered 9 by 5 by 3 inch pan with wax paper.

Sift together the flour, baking powder and salt. Add the fruit and nuts.

Cream the butter and sugar. Beat in the eggs, 1 at a time.

Combine with the fruit and flour mix. Pour into pan.

Bake at 300 degrees Fahrenheit for 1 1/2 to 2 hours or until cake tester comes out clean.

Cool and anoint with bourbon or cognac. Wrap in foil to keep. I usually make these 1 month ahead of when I want to serve them. This is the only fruitcake I ever make.

TANGERINE POUND CAKE

8 servings (Less than 1 mcg of VITAMIN K per serving.)

1	teaspoon	Grated tangerine peel
1	cup	Whipped cream (Stabilized whipped cream will give this dessert a longer shelf life.)
12	ounces	Pound cake, fat free
3 or 4		Tangerines
1/3	cup	Sugar
1	tablespoon	Lemon juice

Stir tangerine peel into whipped cream, chill.

Pierce top and bottom of cake with fork. Place in shallow baking pan. Heat in 350 degrees Fahrenheit oven for 10 minutes.

Peel 2 of the tangerines with a sharp knife, section and seed, reserving segments and juice separately.

Squeeze juice from remaining tangerines to make 1/2 cup.

In saucepan, combine sugar, 1/2 cup tangerine juice and lemon juice. Boil 3 to 4 minutes until slightly thickened, stirring frequently. Slowly spoon hot syrup over bottom, sides and top of warm cake. Let stand 5 minutes.

To serve, slice cake and spoon topping over each piece. Garnish with reserved tangerine sections.

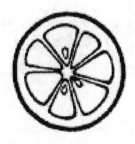

APPLE CAKE

10 servings (1 mcg of VITAMIN K per serving.)

6	medium	Apples peeled and sliced
5	tablespoons	Sugar plus
2	cups	Sugar
5	teaspoons	Cinnamon
3	cups	Flour
3	teaspoons	Baking powder
4	large	Eggs
1	cup	Canola oil, treated (See DIETARY TIP # 10.)
1/4	cup	Orange juice
1	tablespoon	Vanilla
		Whipped cream

Combine peeled apples and 5 tablespoon sugar, add cinnamon.

Sift flour, the rest of the sugar, baking powder and salt into a bowl. Make a well in the center and pour in the oil, eggs, juice and vanilla. Beat with a spoon until blended. Spoon 1/3 of the batter into greased 9 inch angel food pan. Make a ring of 1/2 of the apple mix (drained). Spoon another 1/3 of the batter over apples, spread remaining apples and top with last 1/3 of the batter. Bake in 375 degrees Fahrenheit oven for 1 hour or until done. Test with toothpick. Serve warm or cold with whipped cream.

RASPBERRY WALNUT CAKE

8 servings (7 mcg of VITAMIN K per serving.)

2 3/4	cups	Flour
2 1/2	teaspoons	Baking powder
1/2	teaspoon	Salt
1/2	cup	Unsalted butter (room temperature)
1 3/4	cups	Sugar
1	teaspoon	Vanilla
1/2	teaspoon	Black walnut flavoring
2	large	Eggs (room temperature)
1 1/4	cups	Milk
1	cup	Walnuts, finely ground
1/3	cup	Raspberry preserves
		CREAM CHEESE FROSTING (See Recipe Index)

Preheat oven to 350 degrees Fahrenheit.

Grease and flour two cake pans.

Sift flour, baking powder and salt into bowl.

Using a mixer, cream butter with sugar in another bowl until light and fluffy. Blend in vanilla and walnut flavoring. Beat in eggs, 1 at a time.

Mix in dry ingredients and milk alternately in 3 additions. Fold in 1 cup nuts. Pour batter into pans.

Bake until golden brown and tester inserted in center comes out clean, 30 to 35 minutes. Cool in pans on rack 10 minutes. Turn out onto rack and cool completely.

Heat preserves in heavy small saucepan over low heat, stirring often.

Set 1 cake layer on platter. Spread top of cake with half of preserves. Top with second layer. Spread with remaining preserves. Sprinkle with remaining walnuts.

Spoon 2/3 cup frosting into pastry bag fitted with a star tip, set aside.

Ice sides of cake with remaining frosting. Pipe rosettes of frosting around edge of cake. Refrigerate until frosting is set. (Can do one day ahead.) Let stand 1 hour before serving.

ANGEL FOOD CAKE

8 servings (Less than 1 mcg of VITAMIN K per serving.)

1	cup	Cake flour, sifted
1 1/4	cups	Sugar, granulated, sifted
1	cup	Egg whites at room temperature
1/4	teaspoon	Salt
1	teaspoon	Cream of tartar
3/4	teaspoon	Vanilla
1/4	teaspoon	Almond extract

Sift flour once, measure, add 1/4 cup sugar, and sift together four times.

Beat egg whites and salt with rotary egg beater or flat wire whisk. When foamy, add cream of tartar and continue beating until eggs are stiff enough to hold up in peaks, but not dry. Add remaining 1 cup sugar, 2 tablespoons at a time, beating with rotary egg beater or whisk after each addition until sugar is just blended. Fold in flavoring. Then sift about 1/4 cup of the flour over the mixture and fold in lightly, repeat until all flour is used.

Turn into ungreased angel food pan. Cut gently through batter with knife to remove air bubbles. Bake in slow oven (325 degrees Fahrenheit) 45 to 50 minutes. Remove from oven and invert pan 1 hour, or until cold.

 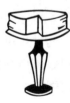 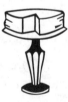 

CHOCOLATE PUDDING CAKE

6 servings (4 mcgs of VITAMIN K per serving.)

CAKE

1	cup	Flour
2	teaspoons	Baking powder
1/2	teaspoon	Salt
3/4	cup	Sugar
2	tablespoons	Cocoa
1/2	cup	Milk
1	teaspoon	Vanilla
2	tablespoons	Mayonnaise, homemade (See Recipe Index)
3/4	cup	Walnuts or pecans, chopped

TOPPING

3/4	cup	Brown sugar
1/4	cup	Cocoa
1 3/4	cups	Hot water

Sift dry ingredients together. Add milk, vanilla and mayonnaise. Mix until smooth. Add nuts. Pour into 9 inch cake pan.

Mix brown sugar and cocoa. Sprinkle over batter. Pour hot water over entire batter. Bake at 350 degrees Fahrenheit for 40 to 45 minutes.

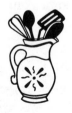

APPLE COFFEE CAKE

9 servings (1 mcg of VITAMIN K per serving.)

2	cups	Flour
1 1/4	cups	Sugar
1 1/2	teaspoons	Ground cinnamon
1 1/4	teaspoons	Baking soda
1/2	teaspoon	Salt
1/4	teaspoon	Ground cloves
1/4	teaspoon	Ground nutmeg
2		Eggs, beaten
1	teaspoon	Vanilla
1/2	cup	Applesauce (replaces 1/2 cup oil)
1/3	cup	Apple juice
2	cups	Chopped peeled apples
1/4	cup	Brown sugar, packed
1/4	cup	Chopped walnuts, optional
		Butter for pan

Sift together flour, sugar, cinnamon, baking soda, salt, cloves, and nutmeg into mixing bowl. Stir to blend.

Add eggs, vanilla, applesauce and apple juice. Stir just until blended. Fold in peeled apples. Spoon batter into a buttered 8-inch square baking pan.

Combine brown sugar and walnuts. Sprinkle evenly over top of batter. Bake at 350 degrees Fahrenheit 40 to 45 minutes or until a toothpick inserted in the center of the cake comes out clean.

RAINBOW CAKES

8 servings (Less than 1 mcg of VITAMIN K per serving.)

2	layers	Cake, white or yellow
3	ounces	Lemon or lime gelatin
3	ounces	Orange gelatin
2	cups	Water, boiling
8	ounces	Whipped cream

Place cake layers top side up, in 2 clean layer pans, prick each cake with utility fork at 1/2 inch intervals.

Dissolve each flavor gelatin separately in one cup of boiling water. Carefully pour one flavor gelatin over one cake layer and the other flavor over the second layer.

Chill 4 hours or more.

Dip one cake pan in warm water for 10 seconds. Unmold, and place on serving plate. Top with 1 cup of whipped cream. Place second layer on top, finish frosting with the remaining whipped cream. (Stabilized whipped cream may be used.)

Chill.

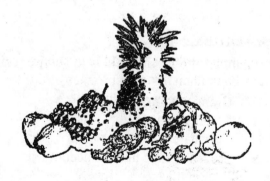

FUZZY NAVEL CHEESECAKE

12 servings (2 mcgs of VITAMIN K per serving.)

COOKIE CRUST

3/4	cup	Flour
2 1/2	tablespoons	Sugar
1	large	Egg, lightly beaten
1/4	cup	Butter, softened
1/2	teaspoon	Vanilla

FILLING

24	ounces	Cream cheese
3/4	cup	Sugar
1/4	cup	Sour cream
5	teaspoons	Cornstarch
3	large	Eggs
1		Egg yolk
1/2	cup	Frozen orange juice concentrate
1/4	cup	Peach schnapps
2	teaspoons	Lemon juice
1 1/4	teaspoons	Vanilla extract

ORANGE MARMALADE GLAZE

1 recipe (Less than 2 mcgs of VITAMIN K in the entire recipe.)

2/3	cup	Orange marmalade
3	tablespoons	Peach schnapps
1 1/2	tablespoons	Cornstarch
1 1/2	tablespoons	Frozen orange juice concentrate
2	teaspoons	Lemon juice

CRUST: In medium bowl, stir together flour and sugar. Add egg, butter and vanilla. Beat with electric mixer until well combined. With greased fingers press dough evenly on to bottom of greased 9 inch springform pan. Bake at 350 degrees Fahrenheit for 12-15minutes or until lightly browned. Remove from oven and set aside.

FILLING: In large bowl combine first 4 ingredients. Beat with electric mixer until smooth. Add eggs and yolk, one at a time, beating well after each addition. Beat in orange juice, schnapps, lemon juice and vanilla. Pour mixture over the crust. Bake at 350 degrees Fahrenheit for 15 minutes. Lower the oven temperature to 200 degrees Fahrenheit and bake for an additional hour and 10 minutes or until center no longer looks shiny or wet. Remove cake from oven and run knife around edge of pan. Chill uncovered, overnight.

GLAZE: In a small saucepan combine all ingredients. Cook and stir until thickened and bubbly. Cook and stir 2 minutes more. Pour over cheesecake. Chill until serving time.

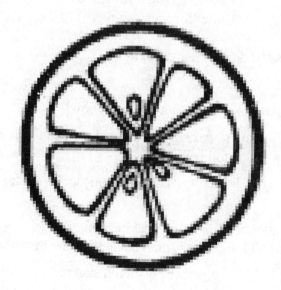

CARROT/ZUCCHINI/APRICOT/PINEAPPLE CAKE

24 servings (3 mcgs of VITAMIN K per serving.)

2	large	Eggs
2		Egg whites
2	cups	Flour
2	cups	Sugar
2	teaspoons	Baking powder
1 1/2	teaspoons	Baking soda
1	teaspoon	Salt
2	teaspoons	Ground cinnamon
1 1/2	cups	Pureed apricots (replaces 1 1/2 cups oil)
2	cups	Carrots, peeled and grated
8	ounces	Crushed pineapple, drained, and the juice reserved
1	cup	Seedless raisins
1/2	cup	Chopped walnuts or pecans,
1	cup	Powdered sugar for glaze
		Butter for greasing pan

Preheat oven to 350 degrees Fahrenheit.

Butter a 9 by 13 inch pan.

Lightly beat together eggs and egg whites in bowl.

Sift together flour, sugar, baking powder, baking soda, salt and cinnamon into mixing bowl. Stir to blend.

Add pureed apricots, beaten eggs, carrots, pineapple, raisins and nuts until blended.

Turn into the buttered 13 by 9 inch baking pan. Bake at 350 degrees Fahrenheit 35 to 40 minutes or until cake tests done in center.

While cake cools, blend together powdered sugar and 2 tablespoons reserved pineapple juice until smooth and of spreading consistency. Drizzle over cake.

Most people look at carrot cake and see a healthy cake. What they forget is that most carrot cakes are made with oil. In the oil version of this recipe there is 1-1/2 cups. But replace the oil with pureed apricots and you reduce the percentage of calories from fat from an extremely high 50% to just 4%. Though they are traditionally added to carrot cake, you may want to omit the walnuts, which are high in fat but are also good for you in so many other ways.

PUREED APRICOTS - 2 cup dried apricots, 3/4 cup water, 2 teaspoon vanilla. Puree apricots, water and vanilla in blender or food processor. Makes 1-1/2 cups

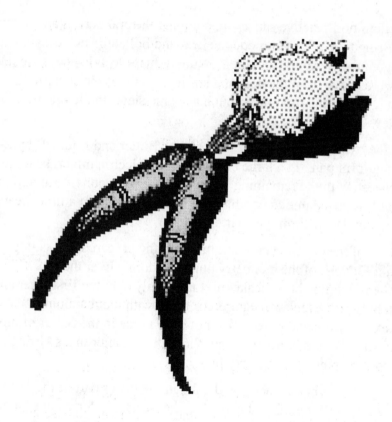

CRANBERRY SWIRL CHEESECAKE

12 servings (2 mcgs of VITAMIN K per serving.)

12	ounces	Fresh cranberries
1 1/3	cups	Sugar
2	tablespoons	Sugar
2	pounds	Cream cheese, at room temperature, cut in pieces
2	teaspoons	Vanilla extract
4	large	Eggs, at room temperature
1	pint	Sour cream, at room temperature

In a medium non-reactive saucepan, combine the cranberries and 3/4 cup water. Bring to a boil over moderate heat and boil, stirring occasionally, until the cranberries burst and the mixture reduces to 1-1/4 cups, about 12 minutes. Remove from the heat and stir in 1/3 cup of the sugar until dissolved. Strain the mixture through a coarse sieve and let the puree cool completely.

Preheat the oven to 275 degrees Fahrenheit. Butter and flour a 9-by-2-3/4 inch springform pan. In a large bowl, using an electric mixer, beat the cream cheese with the remaining 1 cup plus 2 tablespoons sugar and the vanilla at low speed until smooth. Beat in the eggs one at a time, beating until just blended. Stir in the sour cream.

Spoon half of the cream cheese mixture into the prepared pan. Drop 8 or 9 rounded teaspoons of the cranberry puree randomly over the top. Spoon half of the remaining cheesecake mixture evenly over the first layer and dot with half of the remaining puree. Repeat with the remaining cheesecake mixture and puree. (Do not drop puree in the center of more than 1 layer.) With a blunt knife, cut through the batter in a swirling motion to distribute the cranberry puree.

Place the pan on a baking sheet and bake in the lower part of the oven for 1 hour. Turn the oven off and leave the cheesecake in for 1 hour longer. Transfer the cake to a rack and let cool to room temperature. Cover and refrigerate overnight before serving.

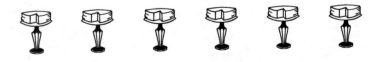

HUNGARIAN COFFEE CAKE

8 servings (3 mcgs of VITAMIN K per serving.)

2	cups	Brown sugar
1	cup	Butter
3	cups	Flour

Using pastry blender, cut shortening into flour and brown sugar until crumbly.

Remove 1 cup of this mixture to small bowl and add 1/8 teaspoon cinnamon and 3 tablespoon white sugar. Set aside for topping.

2	large	Eggs, beaten
1	cup	Buttermilk
1	teaspoon	Salt
1	teaspoon	Baking soda

Beat eggs, add buttermilk and baking soda and salt and mix well. Add remaining flour mixture and beat well with an electric mixer. Turn into two greased 9 inch round pans or one 9x13 inch pan.

Top with crumb mixture and if desired, sprinkle with powdered sugar. Bake at 350 degrees Fahrenheit for 25 to 30 minutes or until done (use toothpick to test).

OPTIONS:

BLUEBERRIES: Sprinkle 2 cups of raspberries with 1/2 cup sugar and lightly toss. Arrange raspberries on top of cake, then sprinkle with crumb mixture. Bake longer (45-50 minutes.) and watch closely at the end. Make sure you bake this longer because of the fruit. (Adds 14 mcgs of VITAMIN K to each cake.)

PEACHES: Peel, pit and thinly slice peaches (about 2 cups), toss with 1/2 cup sugar. Arrange peach slices overlapping on top of cakes, top with crumb mixture. Bake until done (takes longer than regular cake also). (Adds 8 mcgs of VITAMIN K to each cake.)

APPLES: Same as above. Be sure to peel, and slice apples very thin. (Negligible affect on the VITAMIN K content.)

GLAZED BLUEBERRY SHORTCAKE

8 servings (1 mcg of VITAMIN K per serving.)

1/2	cup	Sugar (or to taste)
2	teaspoons	Cornstarch
1/8	teaspoon	Salt
1/2	cup	Water
2	pints	Blueberries, thawed if frozen
1	teaspoon	Grated lime peel
1	tablespoon	Lime juice
1		BISCUIT SHORTCAKE (See Recipe Index)
1	cup	Whipping cream

In saucepan mix sugar, cornstarch, salt and water. Add 1 pint blueberries and bring to boil. Simmer uncovered, stirring until clear and thickened, about 3 or 4 minutes. Remove from heat, stir in lime peel and juice. Cool. Stir in remaining 1 pint of blueberries.

Assemble just before serving.

Whip the cream with 1 tablespoon sugar until soft peaks form.

Spread half the blueberry mix on bottom half of shortcake then spread half of whipped cream. Top with other half of shortcake, remaining blueberry mix and remaining whipped cream.

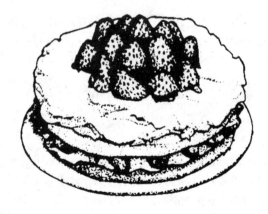

CHOCOLATE HAZELNUT TORTE

6 servings (9 mcgs of VITAMIN K per serving.)

		Unsalted butter and flour for cake pan
1 1/2	cups	Hazelnuts,(filberts) toasted and skinned
1	cup	Granulated sugar
6	ounces	Bittersweet chocolate, finely chopped (6 squares)
4	ounces	Unsalted butter, at room temperature (1 stick)
5	large	Eggs, separated, at room temperature
1/2	teaspoon	Salt
2	tablespoons	Hazelnut liqueur, Frangelico liqueur OR
1	teaspoon	Vanilla, instead of liqueur
		Powdered sugar to dust cake

Place rack in center of oven, preheat to 350 degrees Fahrenheit. Butter and flour a 9 inch cake pan. Line bottom of pan with parchment or wax paper. Butter paper.

In food processor or blender, pulse hazelnuts with 3 tablespoons of sugar until finely ground, about 1 minute. Don't over-process or nuts will turn into hazelnut butter.

Melt together chocolate, butter and remaining sugar, stirring frequently. Beat egg yolks (1 at a time) into chocolate mixture, blending well after each. Blend in liqueur or vanilla. Blend in nut mixture.

Whip egg whites with salt until they hold firm, but not stiff peaks, about 10 minutes. Gently fold whites into chocolate mixture. Pour batter into prepared pan.

Bake 35 minutes, until cake feels firm in center when pressed lightly. Remove from oven and cool cake in pan on rack for 20 minutes. Place a cardboard round or a plate over pan and invert. Remove pan, peel off parchment. Let cool completely. Can be made a day ahead. When cool, wrap completely in plastic wrap and store at room temperature. Dust with confectioners sugar just before serving. (Large strawberries arranged around the cake, on the platter, make a great presentation.)

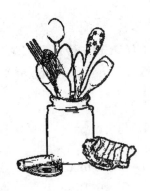

DARK RUM GLAZE

1 cup (9 mcgs of VITAMIN K per cup.)

1/4	pound	Butter
1/4	cup	Water
1	cup	Sugar
1/2	cup	Dark rum

Melt and stir all ingredients except rum over low flame for 5 minutes. Keep stirring and wiping sides of pan. Add rum and use as directed in recipe.

SEVEN MINUTE COFFEE FROSTING

1 recipe (Less than 1 mcgs of VITAMIN K per recipe.)

1	tablespoon	Instant espresso coffee powder
1/4	cup	Hot water
3		Egg whites
1 1/2	cups	Light brown sugar, packed
1	teaspoon	Cream of tartar
1	teaspoon	Vanilla

Dissolve coffee in hot water. Combine egg whites, brown sugar, coffee mixture and cream of tartar in top of double boiler. Beat with mixer until frosting forms stiff peaks, 5 to 7 minutes. Remove from heat. Beat in vanilla. Makes about 5 cups, enough to frost a 2 layer cake or 1 angel food cake.

BISCUIT SHORTCAKE

6 servings (3 mcgs of VITAMIN K per serving without the fruit. If you use a pound of strawberries add 2 mcgs of VITAMIN K per serving. For a pound of blueberries add 5 mcgs per serving. For a pound of peaches add 3 mcgs per serving. For a pound of sweet pitted cherries add 1.5 mcgs per serving.)

2	cups	All purpose flour
1/2	cup	Butter
2	tablespoons	Sugar
1	large	Beaten egg
3	teaspoons	Baking powder
2/3	cup	Milk
1/2	teaspoon	Salt
1	pound	Fruit of choice
		Whipped cream

In a large bowl, sift together the flour, sugar, baking powder and salt. Cut in the butter until the mixture resembles coarse crumbs. Combine egg and milk and add all at once to the dry ingredients, stirring just enough to moisten.

Spread dough in greased 8 by 1 1/2 inch round layer pan, slightly building up edges.

Bake at 450 degrees Fahrenheit oven for 15 to 18 minutes or until golden.

Remove from pan, cool on rack 3 minutes.

With a serrated knife, split horizontally into 2 layers.

Lift top off carefully. Spoon fruit, then whipped cream between layers and then over top. Garnish and cut in 6 wedges.

SEVEN MINUTE FROSTING

1 recipe (Less than 1 mcgs of VITAMIN K per recipe.)

2		Egg whites; unbeaten
1 1/2	cups	Sugar
5	tablespoons	Water
1 1/2	tablespoons	Corn syrup
1	teaspoon	Vanilla
		Boiling water

Combine egg whites, sugar, water, and corn syrup in top of double boiler. Beat with hand mixer or rotary egg beater until thoroughly mixed. Place over rapidly boiling water, beating constantly with mixer or rotary egg beater, and cook 7 minutes, or until frosting will stand in peaks. Remove from boiling water; add vanilla and beat until thick enough to spread. Makes enough frosting to cover tops and sides of 2-9" layers or top and sides of 8 x 8 x 2" cake, generously, or about 2 dozen cup cakes, or top and sides of small angel food cake. To cover top and sides of 3 10" layers, prepare this single recipe twice.

Variations:

Tinted Seven Minute Frosting: Use this recipe and add red, green or yellow coloring to hot frosting to give a delicate tint. Remove from boiling water, add vanilla and beat until thick enough to spread.

Mint Frosting: Use this recipe, using green coloring and 1/4 teaspoon peppermint extract in place of the vanilla. Add coloring gradually to hot frosting to give a delicate tint. Remove from boiling water, add flavoring and beat until thick enough to spread.

DESSERTS

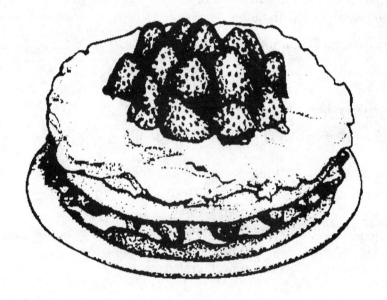

BAKED PEARS IN WINE
2 servings (1 mcg of VITAMIN K per serving.)

2		Firm pears
1/3	cup	Orange marmalade or apricot jam
1/4	cup	Light vermouth
2	tablespoons	Butter

Preheat oven to 350 degrees Fahrenheit.

Peel, quarter and core pears. Cut into 1/2 inch strips. Arrange in two serving dishes.

Mix the marmalade and vermouth in a small bowl and pour this mixture over the pears. Top with butter.

Place in oven and cook for 20 minutes.

KIWI FRUIT ICE
4 servings (22 mcg of VITAMIN K per serving.)

1	cup	Water
1/2	cup	Sugar
1/2	cup	Light corn syrup
1 1/2	cups	Kiwi fruit, pared
5	tablespoons	Lemon juice
1/4	teaspoon	Lemon peel, grated

Combine water, sugar and corn syrup in saucepan. Cook and stir 2 minutes or until sugar is dissolved.

Puree kiwi in food processor or blender to equal 3/4 cup puree. Add lemon juice, peel and sugar mixture.

Pour into shallow metal pan and freeze for approximately 1 hour or until the mixture is firm, but not solid.

When chilled, spoon into a chilled bowl and beat with an electric mixer until the mix is light and fluffy.

Return it to the freezer for approximately 2 hours or until firm enough to scoop.

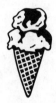 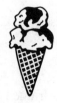 

FRUITY BREAD PUDDING
6 servings (7 mcg of VITAMIN K per serving.)

10	slices	Stale bread
3	large	Eggs, beaten
2	cups	Sugar
1/2	cup	Butter
1	cup	Raisins
1	cup	Pecan pieces
1	cup	Fruit cocktail, with juice
1	can	Pet milk (12 oz)
1	cup	Water
2	tablespoons	Vanilla butternut flavoring

Put everything in a large bowl and mix it.

Turn into a greased 9 by 13-inch pan and bake in a 400 degree Fahrenheit oven for 1 hour and 20 minutes.

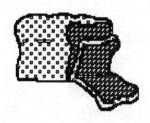

FRUIT COCKTAIL TORTE

9 servings (2 mcg of VITAMIN K per serving.)

1	cup	Flour
3/4	cup	Sugar
1	large	Egg
1	teaspoon	Baking soda
1/4	teaspoon	Salt
1	can	Fruit cocktail(16 oz, drained)
1/2	cup	Brown sugar
1/2	cup	Walnuts or pecans, chopped

Mix all ingredients except brown sugar and nuts.

Place in ungreased 8-inch square pan. Spread top with brown sugar and nuts.

Bake at 300 degrees Fahrenheit for 1 hour. Cool, cut and serve with whipped cream or ice cream.

If you mix this with a fork, the fruit stays whole. If you mix with a beater, the fruit gets chopped. Either way is great.

STRAWBERRIES NAPOLEAN

8 servings (3 mcgs of VITAMIN K per serving.)

PASTRY

2	cups	Sifted all purpose flour
1/2	teaspoon	Salt
1/3	cup	Butter
1/3	cup	Shortening
5	tablespoons	Ice water, approximately

CREAMY STRAWBERRY FILLING

1	pint	Strawberries (or one package frozen)
1/2	cup	Sugar
5	tablespoons	Flour
		Dash of salt
2	cups	Milk

2	tablespoons	Butter
2		Egg yolks
1/2	cup	Whipping cream
1/2	teaspoon	Almond extract

Set oven at 425 degrees Fahrenheit. Sift flour and salt together, then work in butter and shortening. When mixture resembles corn meal, sprinkle water into it, stirring gently but quickly until dough holds together, no more.

Roll out one quarter of the dough on a lightly floured baking sheet to form a thin rectangle 8 by 4 inches. Prick surface several times with a fork. Bake 15 to 20 minutes covered with a sheet of brown paper (to keep edges from getting too brown). Remove from baking sheet and bake the remaining three pieces of dough the same way.

Cut berries in quarters. (When using frozen berries, thaw and drain well.)

Mix sugar, flour and salt in saucepan, stir in milk and add butter. Cook over medium heat, stirring constantly until mix is as thick as a thick custard.

Beat egg yolks slightly, then stir a little of the hot sauce into the egg yolks and add remaining sauce. Cook 2 minutes longer, chill.

Whip cream stiff, then fold gently into the custard along with the almond extract and berries. Spread filling between the 4 layers of pastry, making a stack. To Ice: Beat 2 cups confectioners sugar with 2 tablespoon water and 1/8 teaspoon almond extract. Spread over the top of the stack. Sprinkle with 1/2 cup chopped nuts.

CREME TOPPING

6 servings (Less than 1 mcg of VITAMIN K per serving.)

1	cup	No-fat cottage cheese (or low fat)
2	tablespoons	Skim milk
2	teaspoons	Vanilla
3	tablespoons	Sugar
1/4	teaspoon	Lemon extract

In a blender container, combine all ingredients. Blend until smooth. Chill.

Can be used as a dip for fruit or on top of pies, fruit desserts or cakes.

For a variation try coconut, almond or orange extract in place of the lemon.

FUDGE SAUCE

8 servings (Less than 1 mcg of VITAMIN K per serving.)

3/4	cup	Sugar
1/3	cup	Cocoa
4	teaspoons	Corn starch
2/3	cup	Evaporated skim milk
1	teaspoon	Vanilla

Mix first 3 ingredients together. Then add the milk. Cook until bubbly. Continue cooking for about two minutes. Add Vanilla. Stir and serve.

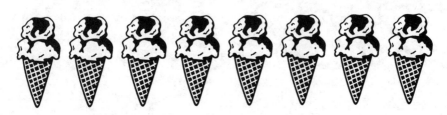

WHIPPED CREAM

2 cups (VITAMIN K content = less than 1 mcg per cup)

1	cup	Whipping cream

Whip the cream until soft peaks form, add 1 tablespoon sugar, if desired. Continue whipping until the cream is stiff.

Cover and refrigerate. When ready to serve, whisk the cream lightly.

STABILIZED WHIPPED CREAM

2 cups (VITAMIN K content = less than 1 mcg per cup)

1	cup	Whipping cream
1	tablespoon	Cold water
1/2	teaspoon	Gelatin, unflavored
1	tablespoon	Sugar (optional)

Whipping cream can be prepared ahead of time by adding gelatin to it.

For each cup of whipping cream, put 1 tablespoon of cold water in a small cup or bowl, stir in 1/2 teaspoon unflavored gelatin and set the cup in a pan of simmering water. Stir until the gelatin dissolves, allow to cool.

Whip the cream until soft peaks form, add the dissolved gelatin and 1 tablespoon sugar, if desired. Continue whipping until the cream is stiff.

Cover and refrigerate for up to 24 hours. When ready to serve, whisk the cream lightly. Note: This is very effective and will hold the whipped cream for several days in the refrigerator.

VANILLA SAUCE

6 servings (Less than 1 mcg of VITAMIN K per serving.)

1 1/2	tablespoons	Butter
1 1/2	tablespoons	Flour or cornstarch
1	cup	Boiling water
	dash	Salt
2	tablespoons	Sugar
1	teaspoon	Vanilla

Melt the butter in a saucepan, stir in the flour or cornstarch and blend well.

Stir in the boiling water, salt and sugar, mixing constantly.

Cook over low heat, stirring constantly, until the mixture thickens.
Remove from heat and add the vanilla.

Serve warm or cold. Serve on cake or apple pie

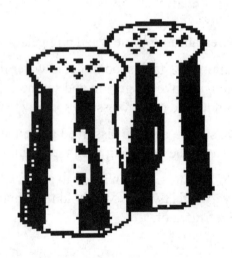

TART APRICOT SAUCE

6 servings (Less than 1 mcg of VITAMIN K per serving.)

8	ounces	Dried apricots
1 1/2	cups	Water
2	tablespoons	Sugar
2	tablespoons	Fresh lemon juice
2	inch	Piece of vanilla bean

Combine apricots, water, vanilla bean and sugar in a 4 cup glass measure. Cover tightly with plastic wrap. Cook in microwave at 100% for 7 minutes in a 650 to 700 watt microwave. Prick plastic to release steam.

Remove from oven and uncover carefully. Drain apricots, reserving juice, and remove vanilla bean. Scrape apricots into a blender. Add lemon juice and puree until smooth. Add as much of the reserved cooking liquid as you wish to get the texture that you like.

You can use glazed apricots for a sweeter sauce. I like it sweeter myself. It is yummy over ice cream, cakes, etc.

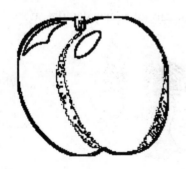

PEACH MELBA TRIFLE

12 servings (3 mcgs of VITAMIN K per serving.)

14	ounces	Sweetened condensed milk
1 1/2	cups	Water
1	package	Instant vanilla pudding mix
1	pint	Whipping cream, whipped
1/4	cup	Plus 1 tablespoon orange juice
10	ounces	Angelfood cake, in small pieces
4	cups	Sliced peaches
1/4	cup	Red raspberry jam, warmed
		Optional: toasted almonds and additional preserves

In a large bowl, combine sweetened condensed milk and water, mix well. Add pudding mix, beat until well blended. Chill 5 minutes.

Fold in whipped cream and 1 tablespoon orange juice.

Place half the cake pieces in a 2 quart bowl. Sprinkle with 2 tablespoons orange juice. Top with half the peach slices, the preserves and 1/2 of the pudding mixture. Repeat layering with remaining cake, orange juice, peaches and pudding. Chill.

Garnish with almonds and additional preserves if you wish.

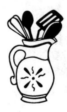

CHOCOLATE BREAD PUDDING

6 servings (Less than 1 mcg of VITAMIN K per serving.)

		Bread, to fill dish 2/3 full
2/3	cup	Sugar
2	tablespoons	Cocoa (heaping tablespoons)
2	cups	Milk
2		Eggs
1	teaspoon	Vanilla

Into a greased casserole dish break up enough bread to fill it 2/3 full. Mix sugar and cocoa and toss lightly with bread.

Add well beaten eggs and vanilla to milk. Pour this over the bread and it should just cover the pieces. Bake at 350 degrees Fahrenheit for about 45 minutes. Serve with milk or with a lump of butter melting into the warm pudding or with whipped cream.

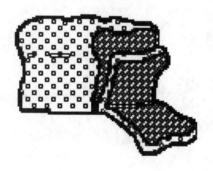

PEPPERED STRAWBERRIES

4 servings (2 mcgs of VITAMIN K per serving.)

1	pound	Strawberries
1	teaspoon	Coarsely ground pepper
4	tablespoons	Sugar
1	tablespoon	Pernod
1	tablespoon	Grand Marnier
4	tablespoons	Heavy cream
2	small	Cantaloupes (or 1 large cut into 4 quarters.)

Wash, dry and hull strawberries.

Sprinkle with pepper. Add sugar and toss gently. Add Pernod and Grand Marnier and toss gently.

Peel cantaloupe, halve and scoop out seeds. Cut down through center, and fan out, and top with strawberry mixture.

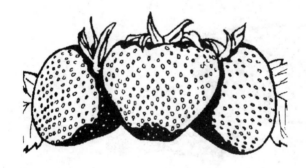

PIES

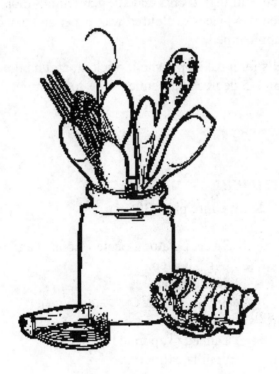

PIE CRUST

One 8 inch two crust pie shell or two single 8 inch pie shells
(12 mcgs VITAMIN K in the entire recipe.)

2 1/4	cups	Flour
1/2	teaspoon	Salt
2/3	cup	Skim milk
3 1/2	tablespoons	Canola oil, treated (See DIETARY TIP # 10.)

For crust, combine all ingredients and stir gently until thoroughly mixed.
Roll out between two pieces of floured wax paper and place in pie plate.
Use as directed in recipe.

If the recipe calls for a baked pie shell, prick all around the shell with a
fork and bake at 375 degrees Fahrenheit for 8 to 12 minutes. Cool and use
as directed.

SWEET POTATO PIE

Total VITAMIN K for entire pie = 30 mcg

3	cups	Sweet potatoes, peeled, cooked and mashed
3	large	Eggs, beaten
1/4	cup	White sugar
1/4	cup	Brown sugar
1/2	teaspoon	Salt
1/4	cup	Canned evaporated skim milk
1	teaspoon	Vanilla extract
1/4	teaspoon	Nutmeg
		PIE CRUST (See Recipe Index.)

For filling, mix all ingredients well.

Pour filling into unbaked pie crust and bake for one hour. Crust will be
golden brown.

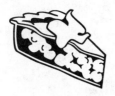

PUMPKIN PIE

8 servings (5 mcgs of VITAMIN K per serving)

1/3	cup	Brown sugar
1/2	teaspoon	Ground cinnamon
1/4	teaspoon	Ground nutmeg
1/4	teaspoon	Salt
1	large	Egg, beaten
3	teaspoons	Vanilla
1	cup	Canned pumpkin
2/3	cup	Evaporated milk
		PIE CRUST (See Recipe Index)

Add all filling ingredients together and thoroughly mix. Pour into prepared pie crust. Bake for 50 minutes at 325 degrees Fahrenheit or until small fork stuck in middle comes out clean.

FUDGE PECAN PIE

8 servings (8 mcgs of VITAMIN K per serving.)

1/3	cup	Butter
1/3	cup	Cocoa
2/3	cup	Sugar
1/4	teaspoon	Salt
3	large	Eggs, slightly beaten
3/4	cup	Light corn syrup
1	cup	Chopped pecans
1	cup	Pecan halves
		Whipped cream
1	8 inch	Unbaked pie crust (See Recipe Index)

Heat oven to 375 degrees Fahrenheit.

Melt butter over low heat, add cocoa and stir until smooth. Remove from heat and cool slightly. Stir in sugar, salt, eggs and corn syrup. Blend thoroughly. Stir in chopped nuts.

Pour into unbaked pie shell. Place pecan halves over top. Bake for 40 minutes. Cool.

Let stand 8 hours before serving. Garnish with sweetened whipped cream.

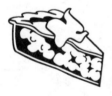 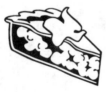 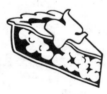

CREAM RAISIN PIE

6 servings (1 mcg of VITAMIN K per serving.)

1	cup	Sour cream
1	cup	Sugar
1	cup	Raisins
1	large	Egg
1	8 inch	Unbaked pie crust (See Recipe Index)

Mix first 4 ingredients thoroughly and pour into unbaked pie shell. Bake at 275 degrees Fahrenheit 90 minutes, until filling is golden brown.

BANANA CREAM PIE

6 servings (Less than 1 mcg of VITAMIN K per serving.)

1	8 inch	Pie crust, baked (See Recipe Index)
1	package	Vanilla instant pudding
1	cup	Milk
1	cup	Sour cream, low-fat
2 or 3		Bananas

Bake pie crust as instructed. Cool.

Make pudding using milk and sour cream.

Slice bananas into pie crust. Cover with pudding. Chill.

Decorate with bananas or whipped cream just before serving if desired.

QUICK & EASY APPLE PIE

6 servings (3 mcgs of VITAMIN K per serving.)

1/2	cup	Flour
3/4	cup	Sugar
		Dash salt
2	teaspoons	Baking powder
1 1/2	cups	Diced peeled apples
1/2	cup	Nut meats
1	large	Egg, beaten
1	teaspoon	Vanilla

Mix together flour, sugar, salt and baking powder and add to peeled apples and nuts.

Beat egg and vanilla. Mix all together. Spread on well oiled 9 inch pie plate.

Bake at 25 minutes at 350 degrees Fahrenheit. Serve warm with vanilla ice cream or with whipped cream.

You can also try half brown and half white sugar.

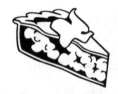

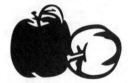

SALADS, DRESSINGS & SAUCES

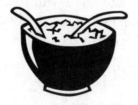

LETTUCE SALAD

1 serving. (Select the ingredients for your salad from the list below. Measure them carefully. Add the number of mcgs (for each of the ingredients selected) together. This will give you the total number of mcgs of vitamin K.)

1	ounce	Iceberg lettuce contains 9 mcgs of vitamin K. (See DIETARY TIP # 16)
1	ounce	Tomato contains 6 mcgs of vitamin K
1	ounce	Carrot contains 5 mcgs of vitamin K.
1	ounce	Cucumber, peeled and sliced, contains 2 mcgs of vitamin K. (Cucumbers must be peeled!)
1	ounce	Onion contains 2 mcgs of vitamin K. (Do not use spring onions!)
1	ounce	Green peppers contains 17 mcgs of vitamin K.

Toss ingredients together and serve with your choice of salad dressings. Don't forget to add the number of mcgs, of vitamin K, in the salad dressing as well. (See Recipe Index.)

ELBOW MACARONI WITH GRAPES

2 servings (15 mcgs of VITAMIN K per serving.)

1/2	pound	Elbow macaroni
1	cup	Green grapes, seedless,
1/4	cup	Celery, sliced
		Salt
1/2	cup	Mayonnaise, homemade (See Recipe Index)
1/2	cup	Sour cream

Whip the mayonnaise and sour cream together, add it to everything else. Serve.

TOMATO AND CABBAGE SALAD

10 servings (VITAMIN K content = 30 mcg per 1/2 cup. Be careful with this recipe! Make certain it is well mixed and each serving contains

proportionate amounts of vegetables. Also, you must weigh both types of cabbage.)

4	ounces	Red cabbage, chopped and carefully weighed (about 1 cup)
2	ounces	Cabbage, chopped and carefully weighed (about 1/2 cup)
2 1/2	cups	Diced tomatoes
1	cup	Sliced radishes
1	teaspoon	Chopped fresh cilantro
1/2	teaspoon	Salt
2	teaspoons	Olive or Canola oil, treated (See DIETARY TIP # 10.)
2	tablespoons	Vinegar or lemon juice
1	teaspoon	Black pepper

Mix all the ingredients in a large bowl.

PIZZA STYLE TOMATO SALAD
8 servings (10 mcgs of VITAMIN K per serving.)

6	large	Tomatoes, thick sliced (approximately 3 cups)
1 1/2	ounces	Pepperoni, thin sliced and diced
5		Pitted black olives, sliced
1/2	cup	Green bell pepper, diced
1/3	cup	Red onions, sliced thin
1	tablespoon	Chopped fresh basil
4	tablespoons	ITALIAN HERB DRESSING (See Recipe Index)
1	cup	Shredded mozzarella cheese
		Salt

Arrange tomatoes on large heat proof platter, slightly overlapping.

Sprinkle with pepperoni, olives, green pepper, onions and basil. Drizzle with dressing, top with cheese.

Just before serving, place under broiler until cheese is barely melted.

CUMIN FLAVORED CARROT SALAD

4 servings (3 mcgs of VITAMIN K per serving.)

1/2	pound	Carrots scraped, ends trimmed
		Chicken broth
		Salt
2	tablespoons	White wine vinegar
1 1/2	tablespoons	Water
1	clove	Garlic, pressed
1/4	teaspoon	Oregano, fresh chopped
1/4	teaspoon	Cumin
1/4	teaspoon	Paprika

Place the carrots in a saucepan with mixture of water and chicken broth to barely cover. Add a little salt. Bring to a boil, cover and simmer for about 10 minutes until just done but still slightly crisp. Cool and cut into 1/4 inch slices.

In a small bowl, mix together the remaining ingredients. Fold gently into the carrots. Marinate for several hours or overnight.

ITALIAN MARINATED TOMATOES

2 servings (14 mcgs of VITAMIN K per serving.)

2	large	Ripe tomatoes
3	cloves	Garlic
1	teaspoon	Balsamic (or other) vinegar
		Salt and pepper

Slice tomatoes into thick slices and arrange them on a plate in one layer.

Chop raw garlic fine and sprinkle over tomatoes. Make sure you get some on each slice! Drop teaspoon of vinegar evenly over tomatoes. (If you like, 3 finely chopped fresh basil leaves can be sprinkled on the tomatoes at this point. This will add an additional 40mcg of VITAMIN K to the entire dish, or an additional 20mcg per serving.)

Let stand at least an hour at room temperature.

Just before serving, salt and pepper to taste. These are good by themselves, on bread, or in a salad.

PINEAPPLE COLESLAW

8 servings (85 mcgs of VITAMIN K per serving.)

DRESSING

1/2	cup	Sour cream, low-fat
1/2	cup	Mayonnaise, homemade (See Recipe Index)
2	teaspoons	Sugar
1	tablespoon	Onion, finely chopped
1	teaspoon	Lemon juice

SALAD

2	cups	Green cabbage, shredded
1	cup	Red apple, peeled chopped
1	cup	Carrots, shredded
3/4	cup	Pineapple tidbits, drained

In small bowl, combine all dressing ingredients, blend well. In large bowl, combine all salad ingredients, toss lightly.

Pour dressing over salad. Mix well.

Cover, refrigerate to blend flavors.

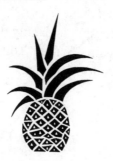

GREEN BEANS CAESAR

8 servings (10 mcgs of VITAMIN K per serving.)

1	pound	Green beans, cooked and chilled
1	teaspoon	Mustard, Dijon
1	tablespoon	Lemon juice
1/2	teaspoon	Worcestershire sauce
4		Anchovies (*or Anchovy paste)
1/2	cup	Olive oil, treated (See DIETARY TIP # 10.)
1	clove	Garlic, minced
1	teaspoon	Pepper, fresh ground
1/2	cup	Parmesan cheese (or 3/4 cup)
1	medium	Egg, raw or coddled (**or use sour cream)
1	cup	Croutons (1 to 2 cups)

*If you use anchovies you need four. If you use the paste it takes more to get the same flavor.

**You can substitute sour cream for the egg if you do not want to eat raw egg.

Put the mustard, pepper, lemon juice, anchovies (or paste), garlic, Worcestershire sauce and 1/3 cup of oil into blender. Puree ingredients.

Taste at this point and adjust seasonings if necessary. Add remaining olive oil, parmesan cheese and egg (or sour cream) to blender. Puree until well blended.

Toss with green beans until dressing is evenly distributed throughout the beans. Add croutons. Toss again. Serve. You can vary the amount of any of the ingredients to suit your own taste.

CUCUMBER "NOODLES" WITH TOMATO SALSA
6 servings (11 mcgs of VITAMIN K per serving.)

| 2 | pounds | Cucumbers, seedless, peeled (about 2 large) |
| 1 | tablespoon | Salt |

FOR THE SALSA

1	pound	Plum tomatoes, peeled, seeded, and chopped
1/4	cup	Onion, finely diced
1	large	Garlic clove, minced
1		Pickled jalapeno pepper, seeded and minced
1	tablespoon	White-wine vinegar
1/4	teaspoon	Sugar

With a sharp knife cut peeled cucumbers lengthwise into 1/8 inch thick "noodles" about 1/2 inch wide. In a bowl toss with salt and let stand for 10 minutes.

Make the salsa while cucumber noodles are standing. Stir together the salsa ingredients.

Drain cucumbers in a colander, rinse under cold water and pat dry on paper towels.

Just before serving, toss to combine.

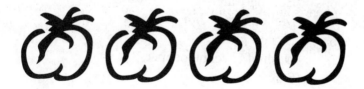

TOMATO AND CUCUMBER SALAD
6 servings (40 mcgs of VITAMIN K per serving.)

2	tablespoons	Fresh ginger root, peeled and minced
2	tablespoons	Fresh garlic, peeled and chopped
1/3	cup	Balsamic vinegar
1	cup	Olive oil, treated (See DIETARY TIP # 10.)
2		Cucumbers, peeled seeded, thinly sliced
15		Roma tomatoes, quartered (approximately 4 cups)
1/4	cup	Scallions, thinly sliced
3		Basil leaves, in thin strips

In a food processor, place the ginger and garlic, and puree them together. With the processor running, slowly add the balsamic vinegar and olive oil. Set the vinaigrette aside.

In a medium large bowl place the peeled cucumbers, Roma tomatoes, scallion, and basil leaves. Mix the ingredients together. Add the vinaigrette and toss it in. Serve the salad at room temperature.

HOLLANDAISE SAUCE
4 servings (3 mcgs of VITAMIN K per serving.)

3		Egg yolks
2	tablespoons	Boiling water
1/2	pound	Melted butter, hot
1	tablespoon	Lemon juice
		Dash of cayenne pepper
		Salt to taste

Put the egg yolks in the electric blender or food processor. If using the blender, turn to low speed. Slowly add the boiling water, and then add the butter very s l o w l y. Add the lemon juice, cayenne and salt. (Usually the butter will have enough salt so be sparing.)

EASY BEARNAISE SAUCE

For an easy Béarnaise sauce cook 1 tablespoon minced shallots with 2 tablespoons vinegar and 1/2 teaspoon fresh tarragon until reduced to a 1 tablespoon. Strain and use this in place of the lemon juice in the HOLLANDAISE SAUCE recipe. (See Recipe Index.)

BERNAISE SAUCE

8 servings or 2 cups (20 mcgs of VITAMIN K per serving.)

1/4	cup	Cider or tarragon vinegar
1/4	cup	Finely chopped onion
1/4	cup	Water or dry white wine
1	tablespoon	Parsley, minced
1	tablespoon	Chives, minced
3		Egg yolks
1/2	cup	Butter
3/4	cup	Mayonnaise, homemade (See Recipe Index.)
1/4	teaspoon	Salt

For meat, fish, seafood, vegetables or meat fondues:

Simmer vinegar and onion until liquid evaporates. Stir in water or wine, parsley and chives and set aside. Beat egg yolks until very thick and lemon- colored. Melt butter. Beat melted butter into egg yolks, a small amount at a time. Turn into heavy saucepan, cook over very low heat, stirring constantly, until thick. Remove from heat and stir in wine mixture. Fold in mayonnaise and salt.

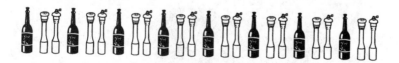

HAND-MADE MAYONNAISE

1 1/4 cups or 20 servings (20 mcgs of VITAMIN K for the entire recipe or
1 mcgs per serving.)

1		Egg yolk
1/2	teaspoon	Salt
1/2	teaspoon	Dijon mustard (or more to taste)
1	tablespoon	Lemon juice or white wine vinegar
1	cup	Light olive oil, treated (See DIETARY TIP # 10.)
		Hot water

Quickly bring the egg to room temperature by setting it in a bowl of hot
water for 2 or 3 minutes, or until the egg no longer feels chilled when held
in your hand.

Then separate out the yolk. Combine the egg yolk, salt, mustard and
lemon juice or vinegar in a bowl. Set the bowl on a folded towel to keep it
from moving around.

Briskly whisk the ingredients together until they are thoroughly blended,
then begin adding the oil, drop by drop at first, then in gradually increasing
amounts.

When the oil is completely incorporated, taste the mayonnaise and add
more salt or lemon juice or vinegar if desired.

A very thick mayonnaise can be thinned by stirring in a spoonful or two of
hot water until you get the consistency you want.

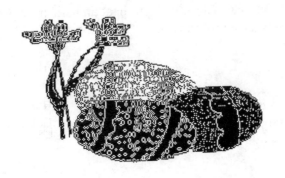

BASIC BLENDER MAYONNAISE

1 1/4 cups or 20 servings (20 mcgs of VITAMIN K per recipe or 1 mcg per serving)

1		Egg
2	tablespoons	Lemon juice
1	teaspoon	Dry mustard
3/4	teaspoon	Salt
1/4	teaspoon	White pepper
1	cup	Oil, olive, treated (See DIETARY TIP # 10.)

Combine egg, lemon juice, mustard, salt and white pepper in a blender or food processor. Cover and blend at low speed until mixed.

Remove center cap. Increase speed to high. Add oil in a thin, s-l-o-w, steady stream. Blend until all oil is added and mayonnaise is smooth and creamy. If necessary, turn motor off and stir occasionally. Replace cover before turning motor back on.

Keep mayonnaise refrigerated and use within 7 to 10 days.

ANOTHER BLENDER MAYONNAISE

1 3/4 cups or 28 servings (28 mcgs of VITAMIN K per recipe or 1 mcg per serving.)

2	Large	Eggs
1	teaspoon	Dry mustard
4	tablespoons	Apple cider vinegar
3/4	teaspoon	Salt
1 1/2	cups	Oil, olive, treated (See DIETARY TIP # 10.)

Blend eggs, vinegar, mustard and seasoning salt in the blender. Add oil very s-l-o-w-l-y (steady flow) while blender continues to run. You may need to stir toward end of adding oil. Makes 1 pint.

TOFU MAYONNAISE

1 1/4 cup or 20 tablespoons (10 mcgs of VITAMIN K per recipe or less then 1 mcg per tablespoon.)

8	ounces	Packed firm tofu, mashed
1	clove	Garlic, minced
1	teaspoon	Dijon mustard
2	teaspoons	Apple cider vinegar
1/2	teaspoon	Salt
1/4	cup	Olive oil, treated (See DIETARY TIP # 10.)

Keeps 1 week in the refrigerator.

Place all ingredients but oil in processor. Process until smooth and creamy, continue to process as you s-l-o-w-l-y drizzle in the oil.

VINEGAR & ONION SALAD DRESSING

1 1/2 cups (12 mcgs of VITAMIN K per recipe.)

1	small	Onion, about 1/2 cup
1/2	cup	Olive oil, treated (See DIETARY TIP # 10.)
1/2	cup	Cider vinegar
1/4	cup	Wine vinegar
3	cloves	Garlic

Put everything in the blender. Process on high for 1 to 2 minutes until pureed. Serve over the LETTUCE SALAD. (See Recipe Index.)

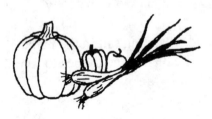

CAJUN MAYONNAISE

2 1/2 cups or 40 tablespoons (1 mcg of VITAMIN K per tablespoon.)

2		Egg yolks
1	teaspoon	Salt
1	clove	Garlic, minced
1/4	cup	Onions, chopped fine
4	dashes	Tabasco sauce
1/2		Juice of 1/2 a lemon
2	cups	Olive oil, treated (See DIETARY TIP # 10.)

Place all the ingredients except the oil in a blender (with the center of the lid removed) or a food processor fitted with a plastic blade and blend or process for 2 minutes.

Pour the oil in a very thin stream, s-l-o-w-l-y, through the top or down the feed tube until it has all been incorporated.

Blend or process for 30 seconds more.

SALSA

4 cups (VITAMIN K content = 11 mcg per cup)

3	cups	Tomatoes, finely cut
1/2	cup	Onion, finely chopped
1	clove	Garlic, finely minced
1/4	cup	Chopped jalapeno peppers
1	teaspoon	Fresh cilantro
		Juice from one lime
1/8	teaspoon	Fresh finely cut oregano
1/8	teaspoon	Salt
1/4	teaspoon	Pepper

Mix all ingredients in bowl. May be served immediately (for best flavor) or after refrigeration.

BASIC VINAIGRETTE

4 servings (2 mcgs of VITAMIN K per serving.)

1	tablespoon	Vinegar or lemon juice
8	tablespoons	Olive oil, treated (See DIETARY TIP # 10.)
1	teaspoon	Salt
1	teaspoon	Dijon mustard
1/2	teaspoon	Freshly ground black pepper

Use your favorite vinegar. Place all ingredients in a jar and shake thoroughly. Add more lemon juice or vinegar to taste. Serve over LETTUCE SALAD. (See Recipe Index)

You can add crushed garlic or Bleu cheese for a different flavor.

BALSAMIC VINAIGRETTE DRESSING

8 servings (VITAMIN K content = 1.5 mcg per serving)

1	teaspoon	Low-fat yogurt
1	teaspoon	Dijon mustard
1/4	cup	Balsamic vinegar
1/8	teaspoon	White pepper
1/3	cup	Olive oil, treated (See DIETARY TIP # 10.)

Whip together all but oil. Add oil s l o w l y, while whipping.

WHITE SAUCE

1 1/4 cup (VITAMIN K content = 3 mcg per cup)

2	tablespoons	Butter
2	tablespoons	Flour
		Salt
		Pepper
1 1/4	cups	Milk, heated

Melt the butter in a sauce pan. Blend in the flour and cook, stirring constantly until thick and starting to bubble. Do not let it brown. Should take about 2 minutes.

Add the hot milk and continue to stir as the sauce thickens. Bring to a boil. Add salt and pepper to taste. Lower heat and cook, stirring constantly, for 2 to 3 minutes more. Remove from heat.

CHEDDAR CHEESE SAUCE

Stir in 1/2 cup grated cheddar cheese during the last 2 minutes of cooking time. (VITAMIN K content = 4 mcg per cup)

MUSHROOM CREAM SAUCE

Stir in 1 cup sliced mushrooms during the last 2 minutes of cooking time. (VITAMIN K content = 3 mcg per cup)

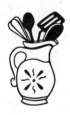

SAVORY WHITE SAUCE

1 1/4 cups (VITAMIN K content = 2 mcg per cup)

2	tablespoons	Butter
3	tablespoons	Flour
1	cup	Hot chicken broth
		Salt
		Pepper

Melt the butter in a sauce pan. Blend in flour and cook, stirring constantly until thick and starting to bubble. Don't let it brown. Should take about 2 minutes. Add the hot chicken broth, continue to stir as the sauce thickens. Bring to a boil. Add salt and pepper to taste. Lower heat and cook, stirring constantly, for 2 to 3 minutes more. Remove from heat.

ITALIAN HERB DRESSING

8 servings (VITAMIN K content = 7 mcg per serving or 56 mcg per cup)

2/3	cup	Olive oil, treated (See DIETARY TIP # 10.)
1/2	teaspoon	Salt
1/2	teaspoon	Fresh oregano leaves
1/2	cup	Wine or white vinegar
1/2	teaspoon	Fresh basil leaves
1/4	teaspoon	Crushed red pepper

Combine all ingredients in a jar. Cover and shake well. Chill to blend flavors. Remove garlic. Shake again before serving. Makes 1 cup.

GREEK SALAD DRESSING

3/4 cup = 8 servings (VITAMIN K content = 56 mcg for the entire recipe
or 7 mcg per serving)

1/2	cup	Distilled white vinegar
1/4	cup	Olive oil, treated (See DIETARY TIP # 10.) and
1/4	cup	Canola oil, treated (See DIETARY TIP # 10.)
1	teaspoon	Fresh oregano
1	clove	Garlic, minced

Simply combine and refrigerate for several days.

HONEY MUSTARD SALAD DRESSING

4 servings (1 mcg of VITAMIN K per serving.)

2	tablespoons	Dijon mustard
2	tablespoons	Honey
2	tablespoons	Mayonnaise, homemade (See Recipe Index)
1/4	cup	Sour cream

Whisk honey and mustard together. Add the last 2 ingredients. At this
point you should taste and add more of whatever you think it needs. May
be used as a salad dressing or as a dipping sauce.

CURTIDO SALVADORENO

10 to 12 servings (VITAMIN K content = 165 mcg per cup)

4	cups	Cabbage, shredded (24 ounces in weight)
1	cup	Grated carrots
1/2	teaspoon	Red pepper
1	teaspoon	Olive oil, treated (See DIETARY TIP # 10.)
1	teaspoon	Brown sugar
1/2	cup	Water
1/4	cup	Vinegar
1	teaspoon	Salt
1/2	teaspoon	Fresh oregano
1/2	cup	Chopped onion

Blanch cabbage in boiling water for one minute. Place cabbage in a container and add the remainder of the ingredients. (Use a fresh 1/2 cup of water.) Refrigerate.

Note: When preparing this recipe, it is essential that the cabbage is actually weighed and 24 ounces used. Also, be aware that this recipe contains a high amount of VITAMIN K and should be consumed accordingly.

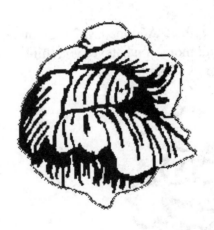

BEVERAGES

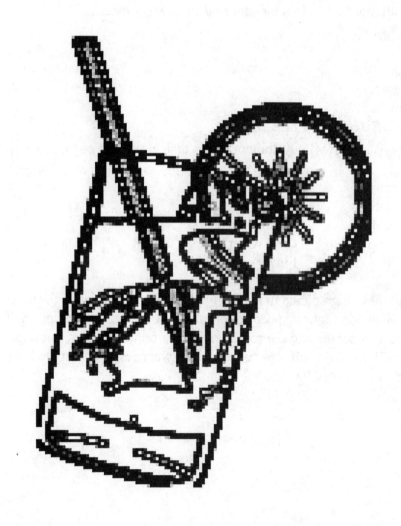

SUMMER FRUIT BLEND
3 servings (VITAMIN K content = 2 mcg per cup)

1	cup	Plain nonfat yogurt
1/2	cup	Strawberries
1	cup	Crushed canned pineapple
1		Banana
1	teaspoon	Vanilla extract
4		Ice cubes

Puree all ingredients in a blender to desired smoothness.

ORANGE JULIUS TYPE DRINK
4 servings (VITAMIN K content = less than 1 mcg per cup)

1/2	cup	Sugar
1	cup	Milk
1 1/2	cups	Orange juice
1	cup	Cold water
1	cup	Finely crushed ice

Add all these ingredients in a 48oz blender, adjust quantities for individual taste. Blend on highest speed for around 5 to 10 seconds and pour. To achieve a closer taste to the real thing use carbonated water, but regular tap water will do. You can also substitute strawberries or pineapple for the orange juice or mix flavors.

FRUIT SMOOTHIE

4 servings (VITAMIN K content = 2 mcg per serving)

8	ounces	Fruit cocktail, can, chilled
1	cup	Milk
1/4	cup	Nonfat dry milk powder
1/2	teaspoon	Vanilla
1/2	cup	Ice cubes
2	dashes	Cinnamon, ground

In a blender container, combine undrained fruit cocktail and remaining ingredients. Cover and blend until combined. Add ice cubes, cover and blend until smooth. Sprinkle with additional cinnamon (for garnish) if desired. Serve immediately.

CIDER SNAP

2 servings (VITAMIN K content is less than 1 mcg per cup)

2	cups	Apple cider or juice
4	teaspoons	Red Cinnamon Candies
4		Thin Apple Slices (Optional)

In a 4-cup measure, combine apple cider and cinnamon candies. Micro-cook, uncovered, on 100% power for 4 to 5 minutes or until candies dissolve and the cider is steaming hot, stirring once. Serve in mugs. Garnish with apple slices if desired.

HOT BUTTERED RUM

2 servings (VITAMIN K content = less than 1 mcg per serving)

2	tablespoons	Brown Sugar
4	teaspoons	Butter, softened
1	dash	Ground Cinnamon
1	dash	Ground Nutmeg
1 1/2	cups	Warm Water
1/2	cup	Rum
		Lemon Slices (Optional)

In a 2-cup measure, stir together the brown sugar, butter, cinnamon, and nutmeg. Stir in the warm water. Micro-cook, uncovered, on 100% power for 3 to 4 minutes or until steaming hot. Stir in the rum. Serve in mugs. Garnish with lemon slices, if desired.

MULLED CIDER

9 (8 ounce) servings (VITAMIN K content is less than 1 mcg per serving)

2	quarts	Apple cider
3/4	cup	Lemon juice
1	cup	Light brown sugar, packed
8		Cloves
8		Cinnamon sticks

In a large saucepan, combine all ingredients. Bring to a boil, reduce heat and simmer uncovered for 10 minutes. Remove spices. Serve hot or cold. Makes two quarts. Note: Some folks have been known to add rum on cold winter days.

BLONDE SANGRIA

6 servings (VITAMIN K content is less than 1 mcg per serving)

1	fifth	Dry white wine
3	teaspoons	Lemon juice
1	cup	Pineapple juice
1/3	cup	Orange juice
1	teaspoon	Lime juice
1/4	cup	Sugar
		Ice cubes
7	ounces	Bottle club soda

Mix all ingredients together. Garnish with lemon and lime slices.

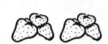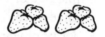

STRAWBERRY SHAKE

2 servings (VITAMIN K content = 1 mcg per serving)

1/2	cup	Strawberries (or more)
2	tablespoons	Honey
1	cup	Cold milk
1	cup	Plain yogurt
2		Whole strawberries

Puree 1/2 cup strawberries and honey in blender or food processor. Add milk and yogurt, blend until smooth. Pour into glasses, garnish each with a whole strawberry. Makes about 2 cups.

PUNCH

20 (4 ounce) servings (VITAMIN K content = less than 1 mcg per serving)

2	quarts	White grape juice
1	quart	Club soda
56	ounces	7-Up

Mix ingredients. Serve well chilled.

RED SANGRIA

12 (6 ounce) servings (VITAMIN K content = less than 1 mcg per serving)

25	ounces	Red wine, dry
1/4	cup	Brandy or cognac
1/4	cup	Triple Sec or Cointreau
1	cup	Orange juice
1	cup	Cider or pineapple juice
1/4	cup	Lemon juice or lemonade concentrate*
1	quart	Club soda or ginger ale
		Sliced citrus fruit
		Sugar as needed (about 1/4 cup)
		Strawberries optional

*Use 1/2 of a 6-oz can of concentrate.
Mix all ingredients, except club soda, refrigerate until chilled. Just before serving, stir in the club soda. Garnish with fruit, if desired.

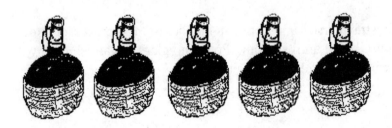

INDEX

A

ALMOND BUTTER COOKIES · 232
AMARETTO CHEESE SPREAD · 47
ANGEL FOOD CAKE · 242
ANOTHER BLENDER MAYONNAISE · 285
ANTIPASTO PLATTER, MIXED · 49
APPLE CAKE · 240
APPLE COFFEE CAKE · 244, 251
APPLE PANCAKE PUFF · 79
APPLESAUCE BANANA BREAD · 84
ARTICHOKE BOTTOMS WITH SHRIMP SAUTÉ · 150
ARTICHOKE DIP · 52
ARTICHOKES
    STUFFED ARTICHOKES · 212
ARTILLERY RACK OF LAMB · 126
ATHENIAN LAMB STEW · 127

B

BABY CARROTS GLAZED WITH BUTTER · 216
BACON AND ONION MUFFINS · 73
BAKED FISH · 148
BAKED HAM WITH PINEAPPLE · 135
BAKED PEARS IN WINE · 258
BAKED PORK CHOPS · 132
BAKED POTATO CHICKEN SOUP- · 170
BAKED POTATOES STUFFED WITH COTTAGE CHEESE · 196
BALSAMIC SQUASH PUREE · 213
BALSAMIC VINAIGRETTE DRESSING · 288
BALSAMIC-GLAZED SALMON FILLETS · 154
BANANA CREAM PIE · 273
BANANA PECAN MUFFINS · 68
BASIC BLENDER MAYONNAISE · 285
BASIC PANCAKES · 81
BASIC VINAIGRETTE · 288
BASQUE PEPPER STEW · 220
BEAN SOUP · 185
BEANS

BEST EVER BAKED BEANS · 220
FRIED GARLIC GREEN BEANS · 215
STRING BEANS, SOUTHERN STYLE · 214
BEARNAISE SAUCE, EASY · 283
BEEF
    BEEF AND LENTIL STEW · 180
    BEEF STIR FRY · 86
    BEEF STROGANOFF · 87
    BEEF TACOS · 89
    CROCK POT CHILI CON CARNE · 90
    ENCHILADA PIE · 92
    GARLIC MEATBALLS · 106
    HAMBURG CASSEROLE · 90
    ITALIAN MEAT LOAF · 103
    MEAT PASTA SAUCE · 199
    MEATLOAF · 88
    OVEN-BAKED BOURGUIGNONNE · 100
    SAUCY MEATLOAF · 95
    STEAK PARMIGIANA · 101
    TEXAS CHILI · 91
BERNAISE SAUCE · 283
BEST EVER BAKED BEANS · 220
BEVERAGES
    BLONDE SANGRIA · 297
    CIDER SNAP · 295
    FRUIT SMOOTHIE · 295
    HOT BUTTERED RUM · 296
    MULLED CIDER · 296
    ORANGE JULIUS TYPE DRINK · 294
    PUNCH · 298
    RED SANGRIA · 298
    STRAWBERRY SHAKE · 297
    SUMMER FRUIT BLEND · 294
BISCUIT SHORTCAKE · 255
BISCUITS
    BUTTERMILK BISCUITS · 69
    CHEDDAR BISCUITS · 64
    CHEDDAR FANS · 67
BLACK CHERRY YOGURT CREAM DIP · 60
BLONDE SANGRIA · 297
BLUE CHEESE
    TANGY BLUE CHEESE DIP · 51
BLUEBERRY BUTTERMILK PANCAKES · 78
BLUEBERRY COFFEE CAKE · 251
BLUEBERRY MUFFINS · 68

BLUEBERRY SHORTCAKE, GLAZED ·
252
BREAD
APPLESAUCE BANANA BREAD · 84
GARLIC BREAD · 80
IRISH SODA BREAD · 83
BREAD PUDDING
CHOCOLATE · 267
BREAD PUDDING, FRUITY · 259
BREADED VEAL CUTLET
(WEINERSCHNITZEL) · 88
BROWN BUTTER ICING · 228
BRUNCH ENCHILADAS · 162
BRUSCHETTA
GRILLED BRUSCHETTA WITH
FRESH MOZZARELLA AND
TOMATOES · 60
BUTTERMILK BISCUITS · 69

C

CAESAR MAYO DIP · 53
CAJUN MAYONNAISE · 287
CAKES
ANGEL FOOD CAKE · 242
APPLE CAKE · 240
APPLE COFFEE CAKE · 244, 251
BISCUIT SHORTCAKE · 255
BLUEBERRY COFFEE CAKE: · 251
CARROT/ZUCCHINI/APRICOT/PINEA
PPLE CAKE · 248
CHEESECAKE · 236
CHOCOLATE HAZELNUT TORTE ·
253
CHOCOLATE PUDDING CAKE · 243
CRANBERRY SWIRL CHEESECAKE ·
250
FRUIT COCKTAIL CAKE · 235
FUZZY NAVEL CHEESECAKE · 246
GLAZED BLUEBERRY SHORTCAKE ·
252
GOLDEN FRUITCAKE · 238
HUNGARIAN COFFEE CAKE · 251
MARBLE CHEESECAKE · 234
PEACH COFFEE CAKE · 251
PUMPKIN-RAISIN CAKE · 237
RAINBOW CAKES · 245
RASPBERRY WALNUT CAKE · 241
TANGERINE POUND CAKE · 239

CANDIED SWEET POTATOES · 206
CANTALOUPE FRUIT SALAD · 57
CAPONATA (EGGPLANT APPETIZER) ·
54
CARAMELIZED CARNITAS · 59
CARROT HORSERADISH SOUP · 181
CARROT POTATO CHOWDER · 182
CARROT VICHYSSOISE · 178
CARROT/ZUCCHINI/APRICOT/PINEAPP
LE CAKE · 248
CARROTS
BABY CARROTS GLAZED WITH
BUTTER · 216
CAULIFLOWER PANCAKES · 216
CAULIFLOWER WITH TOMATOES · 217
CHEDDAR BISCUITS · 64
CHEDDAR CHEESE SAUCE · 289
CHEDDAR FANS · 67
CHEDDAR-ALE CHEESE SPREAD · 46
CHEESE
HAM AND CHEESE PIE · 140
MACARONI AND CHEESE · 197
SPICY BREAKFAST SAUSAGE
CASSEROLE · 164
CHEESE MUFFINS · 69
CHEESECAKE · 236
CHEESY RICE AND HAM · 206
CHICKEN
BAKED POTATO CHICKEN SOUP- ·
170
CHICKEN AND RICE SOUP · 168
CHICKEN BREASTS DIANE · 114
CHICKEN BREASTS WITH DRIED
BEEF · 116
CHICKEN GUMBO · 111
CHICKEN PICCATA · 115
CHICKEN RAGOUT · 108
CHICKEN SAUTÉ BOURGUIGNONNE
inch · 119
CHICKEN SOUP · 169
CHICKEN-FILLED TORTILLAS · 109
CROCKPOT BAKED CHICKEN
BREASTS · 109
HEARTY CHICKEN AND RICE SOUP
· 192
JAMAICAN JERK CHICKEN · 110
LEMON ONION CHICKEN · 113
MARSALA CHICKEN BREASTS inch ·
117
OLD-FASHIONED CHICKEN SOUP ·
168

QUICK CHICKEN CREOLE · 110
RASPBERRY CHICKEN BREASTS · 113
SAUCY HAM AND CHICKEN · 112
SAUTÉED CHICKEN BREAST WITH MUSHROOMS inch · 118
SHERRIED CHICKEN SOUP · 167
CHILI
    CROCK POT CHILI CON CARNE · 90
    TEXAS CHILI · 91
    VEAL CHILI · 97
CHOCOLATE BREAD PUDDING · 267
CHOCOLATE FROSTING: · 230
CHOCOLATE HAZELNUT TORTE · 253
CHOCOLATE PUDDING CAKE · 243
CHOCOLATE WALNUT SQUARES · 227
CIDER SNAP · 295
CLAM
    GARLICKY CLAM DIP · 50
COOKIES
    ALMOND BUTTER COOKIES · 232
    CHOCOLATE WALNUT SQUARES · 227
    FUDGE BROWNIES · 229
    MEXICAN WEDDING COOKIES · 226
    PEANUT BUTTER COOKIES · 228
    PUMPKIN BARS WITH CREAM CHEESE FROSTING · 225
    RAISIN-FILLED BARS · 231
    RUGALA · 224
    SOUR CREAM COOKIES · 232
CORN CHOWDER · 183
CORN MEAL MUFFINS · 72
CRAB
    CRAB DIP · 51
    CRAB-MELT CANAPÉS · 55
    VEAL OSCAR WITH SHRIMP · 96
CRAB DIP · 51
CRACKERS
    POTATO CRACKERS · 80
CRACKERS DEL PASEO · 50
CRANBERRY SWIRL CHEESECAKE · 250
CREAM
    STABILIZED WHIPPED CREAM · 263
    WHIPPED CREAM · 263
CREAM CHEESE FROSTING · 226
CREAM RAISIN PIE · 273
CREAMY BEEF-NOODLE COMBO · 174
CREME TOPPING · 262
CROCK POT CHILI CON CARNE · 90

CROCKPOT BAKED CHICKEN BREASTS · 109
CROSTINI ALLA PORCINI · 62
CROWN ROAST OF LAMB · 124
CUCUMBER "NOODLES" WITH TOMATO SALSA · 281
CUMIN FLAVORED CARROT SALAD · 278
CURTIDO SALVADORENO · 292

D

DARK RUM GLAZE · 254
DATE OR RAISIN BRAN MUFFINS · 71
DEVILED EGGS · 57
DIETARY TIPS FOR THE PATIENT ON COUMADIN® · 27
DIP
    ARTICHOKE DIP: · 52
    BLACK CHERRY YOGURT CREAM DIP · 60
    CAESAR MAYO DIP · 53
    CRAB DIP · 51
    GARLICKY CLAM DIP · 50
    GOLDEN CITRUS-RAISIN DIP · 52
    TANGY BLUE CHEESE DIP · 51
    TIPSY TUNA DIP · 53
DISCLAIMERS · 3
DRIED TOMATO SMOKY SPREAD · 48

E

EARLY BIRD BUTTERMILK PANCAKES · 77
EGG PANCAKES · 70
EGGPLANT APPETIZER, CAPONATA · 54
EGGPLANT CAVIAR · 61
EGGS
    DEVILED EGGS · 57
    ITALIAN EGGS · 163
    SAUSAGE & EGG CASSEROLE · 160
    SCOTCH EGGS · 161
    SPICY BREAKFAST SAUSAGE CASSEROLE · 164
ELBOW MACARONI WITH GRAPES · 276
ENCHILADA PIE · 92

F

FISH
  BAKED FISH · 148
  GRILLED FISH IN FOIL · 158
  MEDITERRANEAN BAKED FISH · 149
  QUICK FISH CHOWDER · 177
  RED FISH CHOWDER · 175
  SOPA DE PESCADO (FISH) · 176
FRENCH ONION SOUP · 190
FRIED GARLIC GREEN BEANS · 215
FROSTING
  BROWN BUTTER ICING · 228
  CHOCOLATE FROSTING: · 230
  CREAM CHEESE FROSTING · 226
  SEVEN MINUTE COFFEE FROSTING · 254
  SEVEN MINUTE FROSTING · 256
FRUIT
  CANTALOUPE FRUIT SALAD · 57
FRUIT COCKTAIL CAKE · 235
FRUIT COCKTAIL TORTE · 260
FRUIT SMOOTHIE · 295
FRUIT SOUP · 188
FRUITY BREAD PUDDING · 259
FUDGE BROWNIES · 229
FUDGE PECAN PIE · 272
FUDGE SAUCE · 262
FUZZY NAVEL CHEESECAKE · 246

G

GARDEN PIZZA · 65
GARLIC BREAD · 80
GARLIC MEATBALLS · 106
GARLICKY CLAM DIP · 50
GAZPACHO · 166
GINGER MUFFINS · 68
GLAZE
  DARK RUM GLAZE · 254
  ORANGE MARMALADE GLAZE · 246
GLAZED BLUEBERRY SHORTCAKE · 252
GLAZED PORK LOIN ROAST · 132
GOLDEN CITRUS-RAISIN DIP · 52
GOLDEN FRUITCAKE · 238
GOLDEN MUSTARD SQUASH SOUP · 194

GOULASH SOUP · 166
GREEK SALAD DRESSING · 291
GREEK-ROAST LEG OF LAMB · 123
GREEN BEANS CAESAR · 280
GREEN CHILE SAUCE · 176
GRILLED BRATWURST · 136
GRILLED BRUSCHETTA WITH FRESH MOZZARELLA AND TOMATOES · 60
GRILLED FISH IN FOIL · 158
GRILLED LAMB AND SAUSAGE KEBABS · 128
GRILLED PORK TENDERLOIN WITH MUSTARD CREAM · 138

H

HAM
  BAKED HAM WITH PINEAPPLE · 135
  BRUNCH ENCHILADAS · 162
  CHEESY RICE AND HAM · 206
  SAUCY HAM AND CHICKEN · 112
HAM AND CHEESE PIE · 140
HAM IN ZIPPY CREAM SAUCE · 140
HAMBURG CASSEROLE · 90
HAND-MADE MAYONNAISE · 284
HERBED RICE TOSS · 205
HOLLANDAISE SAUCE · 282
HONEY MUSTARD SALAD DRESSING · 291
HOT BUTTERED RUM · 296
HUNGARIAN COFFEE CAKE · 251
HUNGARIAN STYLE SOUP · 191

I

IRISH SODA BREAD · 83
ITALIAN EGGS · 163
ITALIAN HERB DRESSING · 290
ITALIAN MARINATED TOMATOES · 278
ITALIAN MEAT LOAF · 103
ITALIAN VEGETABLE SOUP WITH PROSCIUTTO · 171

J

JAMAICAN JERK CHICKEN · 110
JAMBALAYA WITH PASTA · 203
JUMBO POPOVERS · 75

K

KIWI FRUIT GELATO · 258

L

LAMB
  ARTILLERY RACK OF LAMB · 126
  ATHENIAN LAMB STEW · 127
  CROWN ROAST OF LAMB · 124
  GREEK-ROAST LEG OF LAMB · 123
  GRILLED LAMB AND SAUSAGE
    KEBABS · 128
  LEG OF LAMB · 124
  MUSTARD & WINE MARINATED
    LAMB CHOPS · 126
  OVEN-COOKED LAMB STEW · 122
LEMON HERB ROASTED POTATOES ·
  207
LEMON ONION CHICKEN · 113
LEMON PECAN PORK CHOPS · 133
LEMON VEGGIES · 222
LETTUCE SALAD · 276
LIMA BEANS AND SPINACH · 210
LIST OF FOODS WITH VERY LOW
  VITAMIN K CONTENT · 31

M

MACARONI AND CHEESE · 197
MAPLE WHIPPED BUTTERNUT
  SQUASH · 212
MARBLE CHEESECAKE · 234
MARSALA CHICKEN BREASTS inch ·
  117
MAYONNAISE
  ANOTHER BLENDER MAYONNAISE
    · 285
  BASIC BLENDER MAYONNAISE ·
    285
  CAJUN MAYONNAISE · 287
  HAND-MADE MAYONNAISE · 284
  TOFU MAYONNAISE · 286
MEASUREMENT CHART · 43
MEAT PASTA SAUCE · 199
MEATLOAF
  ITALIAN MEAT LOAF · 103
  MEATLOAF · 88
  SAUCY MEATLOAF · 95
MEDITERRANEAN BAKED FISH · 149
MEXICAN WEDDING COOKIES · 226
MINESTRONE SOUP · 192
MIXED ANTIPASTO PLATTER · 49
MOUSSE
  SALMON MOUSSE · 58
MUFFINS
  BACON AND ONION MUFFINS · 73
  BANANA PECAN MUFFINS · 68
  BASIC
    AND VARIATIONS · 68
  BLUEBERRY MUFFINS · 68
  CHEESE MUFFINS · 69
  CORN MEAL MUFFINS · 72
  DATE OR RAISIN BRAN MUFFINS ·
    71
  GINGER MUFFINS: · 68
  ORANGE MUFFINS · 69
  SURPRISE MUFFINS · 69
MULLED CIDER · 296
MUSHROOM CREAM SAUCE · 289
MUSHROOM SAUSAGE PIE · 139
MUSHROOM SOUP · 184
MUSHROOMS
  CROSTINI ALLA PORCINI · 62
  STUFFED · 48
MUSTARD & WINE MARINATED
  LAMB CHOPS · 126
MY RICE-A-RONI · 200

N

NEAPOLITAN PORK CHOPS · 131

O

ODDS AND ENDS · 36
OLD-FASHIONED CHICKEN SOUP · 168

ONE OUNCE (30 GRAMS) FOOD
    MEASURES · 42
ONE POUND (450 GRAMS) FOOD
    MEASURES · 44
ONION PANCAKES · 221
ORANGE JULIUS TYPE DRINK · 294
ORANGE MARMALADE GLAZE · 246
ORANGE MUFFINS · 69
ORANGE SPREAD · 76
OVEN-BAKED BOURGUIGNONNE · 100
OVEN-COOKED LAMB STEW · 122
OYSTERS
    SCALLOPED OYSTERS · 155

P

PAN FRIED TUNA · 146
PANCAKES
    APPLE PANCAKE PUFF · 79
    BASIC PANCAKES · 81
    BLUEBERRY BUTTERMILK
        PANCAKES · 78
    EARLY BIRD BUTTERMILK
        PANCAKES · 77
    EGG PANCAKES · 70
    ONION PANCAKES · 221
    RICE PANCAKES · 72
PASTA
    MACARONI AND CHEESE · 197
    MEAT PASTA SAUCE · 199
    MY RICE-A-RONI · 200
    PASTA AND TURKEY MEAT RED
        SAUCE · 198
    PASTA JAMBALAYA · 203
    POLISH NOODLES AND CABBAGE ·
        204
    QUICK TOMATO SAUCE FOR PASTA
        · 200
    SHRIMP AND WINE-SAUCED
        SPAGHETTI · 202
PATE
    SALMON AND GOUDA PATE · 56
PEACH COFFEE CAKE: · 251
PEACH MELBA TRIFLE · 266
PEACHY PORK CHOPS · 130
PEANUT BUTTER COOKIES · 228
PEANUT PORK CHOPS · 136
PEARS
    BAKED PEARS IN WINE · 258

PEPPER GRILLED SALMON · 147
PEPPERED STRAWBERRIES · 268
PEPPERS
    BASQUE PEPPER STEW · 220
    STUFFED PEPPERS · 218
PIE CRUST · 270
PIES
    CREAM RAISIN PIE · 273
    FUDGE PECAN PIE · 272
    PUMPKIN PIE · 271
    QUICK & EASY APPLE PIE · 274
    SWEET POTATO PIE · 270
PINEAPPLE COLESLAW · 279
PINEAPPLE YAM BAKE · 222
PISTACHIO-BASIL BUTTER, SALMON
    WITH · 156
PIZZA
    GARDEN PIZZA · 65
    SAUSAGE, EGGPLANT, BASIL AND
        TOMATO PIZZA · 74
    UPSIDE DOWN PIZZA · 104
PIZZA DOUGH: · 66
PIZZA STYLE TOMATO SALAD · 277
POLENTA · 201
POPOVERS
    JUMBO POPOVERS · 75
PORK
    BAKED PORK CHOPS · 132
    CARMELIZED CARNITAS · 59
    GLAZED PORK LOIN ROAST · 132
    GRILLED PORK TENDERLOIN WITH
        MUSTARD CREAM · 138
    LEMON PECAN PORK CHOPS · 133
    NEAPOLITAN PORK CHOPS · 131
    PEACHY PORK CHOPS · 130
    PEANUT PORK CHOPS · 136
    PORK CHOPS BRAISED WITH CIDER
        AND APPLES · 130
    PORK CHOPS IN TOMATO SAUCE
        WITH OREGANO · 144
    PORK CHOPS PARMESAN · 142
    PORK CHOPS WITH ONIONS · 137
    PORK LOIN WITH MUSTARD CRUST
        · 141
    PORK MARENGO · 143
    PORK PINWHEELS WITH APRICOT
        STUFFING · 134
POTATO CRACKERS · 80
POTATO SOUP · 187
POTATOES

BAKED POTATOES STUFFED WITH
COTTAGE CHEESE · 196
CANDIED SWEET POTATOES · 206
LEMON HERB ROASTED POTATOES
· 207
POTATO CASSEROLE · 208
RAW POTATO LOAF · 197
PUMPKIN BARS WITH CREAM
CHEESE FROSTING · 225
PUMPKIN PIE · 271
PUMPKIN-RAISIN CAKE · 237
PUNCH · 298
PUREE OF CARROT SOUP · 180

Q

QUICK AND EASY APPLE PIE · 274
QUICK AND EASY ROLLS · 70
QUICK CHICKEN CREOLE · 110
QUICK FISH CHOWDER · 177
QUICK TOMATO SAUCE FOR PASTA ·
200

R

RAINBOW CAKES · 245
RAISIN
GOLDEN CITRUS-RAISIN DIP · 52
RAISIN-FILLED BARS · 231
RASPBERRY CHICKEN BREASTS · 113
RASPBERRY WALNUT CAKE · 241
RAW POTATO LOAF · 197
RED FISH CHOWDER · 175
RED SANGRIA · 298
RICE
CHEESY RICE AND HAM · 206
HERBED RICE TOSS · 205
MY RICE-A-RONI · 200
RICE PANCAKES · 72
TASTY WHITE RICE WITH CORN ·
196
RICE PANCAKES · 72
ROAST TURKEY · 120
ROLLS
QUICK AND EASY ROLLS · 70
RUGALA · 224

S

SALAD DRESSING
BALSAMIC VINAIGRETTE
DRESSING · 288
BASIC VINAIGRETTE · 288
GREEK SALAD DRESSING · 291
HONEY MUSTARD SALAD
DRESSING · 291
ITALIAN HERB DRESSING · 290
VINEGAR & ONION SALAD
DRESSING · 286
SALADS
CUCUMBER "NOODLES" WITH
TOMATO SALSA · 281
CUMIN FLAVORED CARROT SALAD
· 278
CURTIDO SALVADORENO · 292
ELBOW MACARONI WITH GRAPES ·
276
GREEN BEANS CAESAR · 280
ITALIAN MARINATED TOMATOES ·
278
LETTUCE SALAD · 276
PINEAPPLE COLESLAW · 279
PIZZA STYLE TOMATO SALAD · 277
TOMATO AND CABBAGE SALAD ·
276
TOMATO AND CUCUMBER SALAD ·
282
SALMON
BAKED SALMON WITH FETA
VINAIGRETTE · 157
BALSAMIC-GLAZED SALMON
FILLETS · 154
PEPPER GRILLED SALMON · 147
SALMON AND GOUDA PATE · 56
SALMON GRILL DIABLE · 151
SALMON MOUSSE · 58
SALMON WITH PISTACHIO-BASIL
BUTTER · 156
SEAFOOD STROGANOFF · 153
SMOKED SALMON-AND-CHIVE
SANDWICHES · 75
SALSA · 287
SANDWICHES
SMOKED SALMON-AND-CHIVE
SANDWICHES · 75
TUNA BUNS · 76
SAUCE

BERNAISE SAUCE · 283
CHEDDAR CHEESE SAUCE · 289
EASY BEARNAISE SAUCE · 283
FUDGE SAUCE · 262
GREEN CHILE SAUCE · 176
HOLLANDAISE SAUCE · 282
MUSHROOM CREAM SAUCE · 289
SAVORY WHITE SAUCE · 290
TART APRICOT SAUCE · 265
TURKEY SPAGHETTI SAUCE · 115
VANILLA SAUCE · 264
WHITE SAUCE · 289
SAUCY HAM AND CHICKEN · 112
SAUCY MEATLOAF · 95
SAUSAGE
GRILLED BRATWURST · 136
GRILLED LAMB AND SAUSAGE
KEBABS · 128
MUSHROOM SAUSAGE PIE · 139
SAUSAGE & EGG CASSEROLE · 160
SAUSAGE CHOWDER · 182
SAUSAGE, EGGPLANT, BASIL AND
TOMATO PIZZA · 74
SPICY BREAKFAST SAUSAGE
CASSEROLE · 164
SAUTÉED CHICKEN BREAST WITH
MUSHROOMS · 118
SAUTÉED GARLIC SHRIMP · 146
SAVORY WHITE SAUCE · 290
SCALLOPED OYSTERS · 155
SCONES
SCOTTISH SCONES · 82
SCOTCH EGGS · 161
SCOTTISH SCONES · 82
SEAFOOD STROGANOFF · 153
SEVEN MINUTE COFFEE FROSTING ·
254
SEVEN MINUTE FROSTING · 256
SHERRIED CHICKEN SOUP · 167
SHRIMP
ARTICHOKE BOTTOMS WITH
SHRIMP SAUTÉ · 150
SAUTÉED GARLIC SHRIMP · 146
SEAFOOD STROGANOFF · 153
SHRIMP AND WINE-SAUCED
SPAGHETTI · 202
SHRIMP SPREAD · 46
SHRIMP WITH TOMATO SAUCE · 152
VEAL OSCAR WITH SHRIMP · 96
SMOKED SALMON-AND-CHIVE
SANDWICHES · 75

SMOTHERED GREENS · 210
SOPA DE PESCADO (FISH) · 176
SOUP
BAKED POTATO CHICKEN SOUP- ·
170
BEAN SOUP · 185
BEEF AND LENTIL STEW · 180
CARROT HORSERADISH SOUP · 181
CARROT POTATO CHOWDER · 182
CARROT VICHYSSOISE · 178
CHICKEN AND RICE SOUP · 168
CHICKEN SOUP · 169
CORN CHOWDER · 183
CREAMY BEEF-NOODLE COMBO ·
174
FRENCH ONION SOUP · 190
FRUIT SOUP · 188
GAZPACHO · 166
GOLDEN MUSTARD SQUASH SOUP ·
194
GOULASH SOUP · 166
HEARTY CHICKEN AND RICE SOUP
· 192
HUNGARIAN STYLE SOUP · 191
ITALIAN VEGETABLE SOUP WITH
PROSCIUTTO · 171
MINESTRONE SOUP · 192
MUSHROOM SOUP · 184
OLD-FASHIONED CHICKEN SOUP ·
168
POTATO SOUP · 187
PUREE OF CARROT SOUP · 180
QUICK FISH CHOWDER · 177
RED FISH CHOWDER · 175
SAUSAGE CHOWDER · 182
SHERRIED CHICKEN SOUP · 167
SOPA DE PESCADO (FISH) · 176
STRAW MUSHROOM SOUP · 186
SWEET SQUASH BISQUE · 188
TEX-MEX BEEF SOUP · 173
TOMATO BISQUE · 178
TOMATO SOUP · 189
TOMATO-BEEF SOUP · 172
VEGETABLE SOUP · 179
VEGETABLE-BEEF SOUP · 174
WHITE GAZPACHO · 186
WINTER SQUASH, APPLE AND
WALNUT SOUP · 193
SOUR CREAM COOKIES · 232
SPICY BREAKFAST SAUSAGE
CASSEROLE · 164

SPINACH
LIMA BEANS AND SPINACH · 210
SPREAD
AMARETTO CHEESE SPREAD · 47
CHEDDAR-ALE CHEESE SPREAD · 46
DRIED TOMATO SMOKY SPREAD · 48
ORANGE SPREAD · 76
SHRIMP SPREAD · 46
SQUASH
BALSAMIC SQUASH PUREE · 213
SUMMER SQUASH STIR-FRY · 214
STABILIZED WHIPPED CREAM · 263
STEAK PARMIGIANA · 101
STIR FRY
BEEF · 86
STRAW MUSHROOM SOUP · 186
STRAWBERRIES
PEPPERED STRAWBERRIES · 268
STRAWBERRIES NAPOLEAN · 260
STRAWBERRY SHAKE · 297
STRING BEANS, SOUTHERN STYLE · 214
STROGANOFF
BEEF · 87
SEAFOOD STROGANOFF · 153
STUFFED ARTICHOKES · 212
STUFFED MUSHROOMS · 48
STUFFED PEPPERS · 218
SUBSTITUTIONS · 39
SUCCOTASH · 211
SUMMER FRUIT BLEND · 294
SUMMER SQUASH STIR-FRY · 214
SURPRISE MUFFINS · 69
SWEET POTATO PIE · 270
SWEET POTATOES, CANDIED · 206
SWEET SQUASH BISQUE · 188

T

TANGERINE POUND CAKE · 239
TANGY BLUE CHEESE DIP · 51
TART APRICOT SAUCE · 265
TASTY WHITE RICE WITH CORN · 196
TEAR OUT - LIST OF FOODS WITH VERY LOW VITAMIN K CONTENT · 315, 317
TEXAS CHILI · 91

TEX-MEX BEEF SOUP · 173
TIPSY TUNA DIP · 53
TOFU MAYONNAISE · 286
TOMATO AND CABBAGE SALAD · 276
TOMATO AND CUCUMBER SALAD · 282
TOMATO BISQUE · 178
TOMATO SOUP · 189
TOMATO-BEEF SOUP · 172
TOMATOES
QUICK TOMATO SAUCE FOR PASTA · 200
TORTE
FRUIT COCKTAIL TORTE · 260
TRIFLE
PEACH MELBA TRIFLE · 266
TUNA
PAN FRIED TUNA · 146
TUNA BUNS · 76
TURKEY
PASTA AND TURKEY MEAT RED SAUCE · 198
ROAST TURKEY · 120
TURKEY SPAGHETTI SAUCE · 115

U

UPSIDE DOWN PIZZA · 104
USEFUL DIETARY TIPS FOR THE PATIENT ON COUMADIN® · 27
USEFUL INFORMATION FOR THE COOK · 35

V

VANILLA SAUCE · 264
VEAL
BREADED VEAL CUTLET (WEINERSCHNITZEL) · 88
VEAL CHILI · 97
VEAL MARSALA · 94
VEAL NORMANDE · 94
VEAL OSCAR WITH SHRIMP · 96
VEAL PARMIGIANA · 93
VEAL PICCATA · 98
VEAL SALTIMBOCCA ALLA ROMANA · 102
VEAL SCALOPPINI · 99

VEGETABLE SOUP · 179
VEGETABLE-BEEF SOUP · 174
VEGETABLES
  BABY CARROTS GLAZED WITH
    BUTTER · 216
  BALSAMIC SQUASH PUREE · 213
  BASQUE PEPPER STEW · 220
  BEST EVER BAKED BEANS · 220
  CAULIFLOWER PANCAKES · 216
  CAULIFLOWER WITH TOMATOES ·
    217
  FRIED GARLIC GREEN BEANS · 215
  LEMON VEGGIES · 222
  LIMA BEANS AND SPINACH · 210
  MAPLE WHIPPED BUTTERNUT
    SQUASH · 212
  ONION PANCAKES · 221
  SMOTHERED GREENS · 210
  STRING BEANS, SOUTHERN STYLE ·
    214
  STUFFED ARTICHOKES · 212
  STUFFED PEPPERS · 218
  SUCCOTASH · 211
  SUMMER SQUASH STIR-FRY · 214
  VEGETABLE STEW · 211

ZUCCHINI AND CHEDDAR BAKE ·
  217
ZUCCHINI CASSEROLE · 218
ZUCCHINI-TOMATO PIE · 219
VERMONT CHEDDAR AND MAPLE
  CRACKERS · 49
VINEGAR & ONION SALAD DRESSING
  · 286

W

WHIPPED CREAM · 263
WHITE GAZPACHO · 186
WHITE SAUCE · 289
WINTER SQUASH, APPLE AND
  WALNUT SOUP · 193

Z

ZUCCHINI CASSEROLE · 218
ZUCCHINI-TOMATO PIE · 219

Order Form

✳ **Fax orders: (410) 749-9054**

(**Telephone orders: Call: (410) 749-1989. Have your VISA, Mastercard, Discover or AMEX card ready.**

☂ **Postal orders: Marsh Publishing Company, PO Box 1597, Salisbury, MD 21802-1597, USA**

Please send me _____ copies of the COUMADIN® Cookbook at $16.95 per copy, plus handling, to:

Name:_____.

Address:_____.

City:_____State:_____Zip:_____.

Telephone: (_____)_____-_____.

I understand that I may return any books for a full refund, less shipping and handling, for any reason, no questions asked.

Sales tax:
Please add 5% sales tax for books shipped to Maryland addresses.

Handling:
$4.00 for the first book and $2.00 for each additional book to the same address.

Payment:
☐ **Cheque or Money order**

☐ **Credit card: ☐ VISA, ☐ MasterCard, ☐ Discover, ☐ AMEX**

Card number:_____

Name on card:_____Exp. Date:_____

Order Form

Please send me _____ copies of the **COUMADIN® Cookbook** at $16.95 per copy, plus handling, to:

Name:_____.

Address:_____.

City:_____**State:**_____**Zip:**_____.

Telephone: (_____)_____-_____.

I understand that I may return any books for a full refund, less shipping and handling, for any reason, no questions asked.

Sales tax:
Please add 5% sales tax for books shipped to Maryland addresses.

Handling:
$4.00 for the first book and $2.00 for each additional book to the same address.

Payment:

☐ **Cheque or Money order**

☐ **Credit card: ☐ VISA, ☐ MasterCard, ☐ Discover, ☐ AMEX**

Card number:_____

Name on card:_____**Exp. Date:**_____

Order Form

---

*   **Fax orders: (410) 749-9054**

(**Telephone orders: Call: (410) 749-1989. Have your VISA, Mastercard, Discover or AMEX card ready.**

   Postal orders: Marsh Publishing Company, PO Box 1597, Salisbury, MD 21802-1597, USA

Please send me _____ copies of the **COUMADIN® Cookbook** at $16.95 per copy, plus handling, to:

Name:_____.

Address:_____.

City:_____**State:**_____**Zip:**_____.

Telephone: (_____)_____-_____.

I understand that I may return any books for a full refund, less shipping and handling, for any reason, no questions asked.

Sales tax:
Please add 5% sales tax for books shipped to Maryland addresses.

Handling:
$4.00 for the first book and $2.00 for each additional book to the same address.

Payment:
☐   **Cheque or Money order**

☐   **Credit card: ☐ VISA, ☐ MasterCard, ☐ Discover, ☐ AMEX**

Card number:_____

Name on card:_____Exp. Date:_____

TEAR OUT - LIST OF FOODS WITH VERY LOW VITAMIN K CONTENT

This section is the listing of foods with very little vitamin K content for you to cut out and carry with you. With this list, the patient on COUMADIN® can put into their diet any of the foods listed with little effect on their overall vitamin K intake. The criteria used to place a food on the list below was that it had to contain less than 2 mcgs of vitamin K per 100 grams (approximately 3 1/2 ounces) or milliliters.

- Apple juice
- Apple sauce
- Apple, skinless
- Bagel, plain
- Baking powder
- Banana
- Barley products (flour, bread)
- Beef
- Black olives
- Black pepper
- Bran flakes
- Bread (white, corn, or wheat)
- Cake (angel food)
- Chicken
- Coffee (caffeinated and decaffeinated)
- Cola
- Corn
- Corn flakes
- Corn oil
- Crackers (graham, wheat, or saltine, but watch out for additives, especially oils)
- Cranberry products (juice, sauce, etc.)
- Cream (note: for every one per cent of fat in a milk product, there is only one-tenth of one microgram of vitamin K per 100 grams or 100 milliliters)
- Cucumber, skinless
- Eel
- Egg white
- Egg yolk
- Eggplant
- Garlic and garlic powder
- Ginger ale
- Grapefruit, grapefruit juice
- Grapes, grape juice, grape jelly, etc.
- Honey
- Ice cream
- Jell-O
- Lemon juice, lemonade (the real stuff- not that artificial junk)
- Lemon peel
- Melon, cantaloupe
- Milk (see note above for "Cream")
- Millet
- Mushrooms
- Octopus
- Onions (but NOT spring onions)

- Oranges, orange juice
- Oysters
- Parsnips
- Peaches (canned)
- Peanuts (but NOT peanut butter)
- Pears (canned)
- Pineapple, pineapple juice
- Pork
- Pretzels
- Prunes, prune juice
- Radishes
- Raisins
- Rice, puffed rice, rice flour
- Sake
- Salmon
- Salt
- Sardine
- Shrimp
- Spaghetti
- Squid
- Sugar
- Tea, brewed (black only-not green)
- Tofu
- Turkey
- Turnips
- Vanilla
- Vinegar
- Wheat flour, wheat bread, puffed wheat, shredded wheat
- Wine
- Yellowtail (snapper)
- Yogurt, plain only

Some very common foods just missed making the list above. These include:
- Potato products which contain, when cooked, 10 micrograms (mcgs) of vitamin K per 100 grams,
- Tomato and tomato products (4 to 7 mcgs per 100 grams)
- Celery (12 micrograms per 100 grams)
- Cheddar cheese (3 micrograms per 100 grams)
- Oatmeal (3 micrograms per 100 grams)
- Peanut butter (10 micrograms per 100 grams)
- Squash (3 micrograms per 100 grams)

TEAR OUT - LIST OF FOODS WITH VERY LOW VITAMIN K CONTENT

This section is the listing of foods with very little vitamin K content for you to cut out and carry with you. With this list, the patient on COUMADIN® can put into their diet any of the foods listed with little effect on their overall vitamin K intake. The criteria used to place a food on the list below was that it had to contain less than 2 mcgs of vitamin K per 100 grams (approximately 3 1/2 ounces) or milliliters.

- Apple juice
- Apple sauce
- Apple, skinless
- Bagel, plain
- Baking powder
- Banana
- Barley products (flour, bread)
- Beef
- Black olives
- Black pepper
- Bran flakes
- Bread (white, corn, or wheat)
- Cake (angel food)
- Chicken
- Coffee (caffeinated and decaffeinated)
- Cola
- Corn
- Corn flakes
- Corn oil
- Crackers (graham, wheat, or saltine, but watch out for additives, especially oils)
- Cranberry products (juice, sauce, etc.)
- Cream (note: for every one per cent of fat in a milk product, there is only one-tenth of one microgram of vitamin K per 100 grams or 100 milliliters)
- Cucumber, skinless
- Eel
- Egg white
- Egg yolk
- Eggplant
- Garlic and garlic powder
- Ginger ale
- Grapefruit, grapefruit juice
- Grapes, grape juice, grape jelly, etc.
- Honey
- Ice cream
- Jell-O
- Lemon juice, lemonade (the real stuff- not that artificial junk)
- Lemon peel
- Melon, cantaloupe
- Milk (see note above for "Cream")
- Millet
- Mushrooms
- Octopus
- Onions (but NOT spring onions)

- Oranges, orange juice
- Oysters
- Parsnips
- Peaches (canned)
- Peanuts (but NOT peanut butter)
- Pears (canned)
- Pineapple, pineapple juice
- Pork
- Pretzels
- Prunes, prune juice
- Radishes
- Raisins
- Rice, puffed rice, rice flour
- Sake
- Salmon
- Salt
- Sardine
- Shrimp
- Spaghetti
- Squid
- Sugar
- Tea, brewed (black only-not green)
- Tofu
- Turkey
- Turnips
- Vanilla
- Vinegar
- Wheat flour, wheat bread, puffed wheat, shredded wheat
- Wine
- Yellowtail (snapper)
- Yogurt, plain only

Some very common foods just missed making the list above. These include:

- Potato products which contain, when cooked, 10 micrograms (mcgs) of vitamin K per 100 grams,
- Tomato and tomato products (4 to 7 mcgs per 100 grams)
- Celery (12 micrograms per 100 grams)
- Cheddar cheese (3 micrograms per 100 grams)
- Oatmeal (3 micrograms per 100 grams)
- Peanut butter (10 micrograms per 100 grams)
- Squash (3 mcg per 100 grams)